14-DAY

HERBAL

CLEANSING

14-DAY

HERBAL

CLEANSING

LAUREL VUKOVIC

PRENTICE HALL
Paramus, New Jersey 07652

Library of Congress Cataloging-in-Publication Data

Vukovic, Laurel.
    14-day herbal cleansing / by Laurel Vukovic.
       p. cm.
    Includes index.
    ISBN 0-13-602582-X (preprinted case).—ISBN 0-13-602574-9 (paper)
    1. Herbs—Therapeutic use. 2. Toxins. 3. Health. I. Title.
    RM666.H33VV85 1998   97-40455
    615'.321—dc21   CIP

Printed in the United States of America

10 9 8 7 6 5 4 3 2   10 9 8 7 6 5   (p)

ISBN 0-13-602582-X (preprinted case)

ISBN 0-13-602574-9 (paper)

ATTENTION: CORPORATIONS AND SCHOOLS

Prentice Hall books are available at quantity discounts with bulk purchase for educational, business, or sales promotional use. For information, please write to: Prentice Hall Special Sales, 240 Frisch Court, Paramus, New Jersey 07652. Please supply: title of book, ISBN number, quantity, how the book will be used, date needed.

PRENTICE HALL
Paramus, NJ 07652

On the World Wide Web at http://www.phdirect.com

DEDICATION

Be fully who you are,
for there will never again be anyone like you.

ACKNOWLEDGMENTS

There are many people who have touched my life and have helped to make this book possible. I am especially grateful to:

My mother and father, for their love and enthusiastic support.

My friend and teacher, Rosemary Gladstar, who always inspires me with her heartfelt teachings in the ways of herbalism.

The wonderful editorial staff at Natural Health magazine, with whom I've been privileged to be associated with for the past six years.

Doug Corcoran, my editor at Prentice Hall, for giving me the opportunity to write this book and for being so incredibly patient, and Jackie Roulette for making the production so effortless.

My students, who delight me and from whom I learn so much.

My dear friends who have loved, encouraged, and supported me through the birthing of this book, many of whom have shared long early morning walks with me.

Christopher Briscoe, for his great photography.

And Dragan, for always believing in me.

Table of Contents

PART ONE
Cleansing: The Key to Optimal Health

1

PART TWO
Your Body's Pathways of Detoxification
67

PART THREE
Creating a Cleansing Program
113

chapter fourteen   184
Exercise to Increase Detoxification

chapter fifteen   201
The Healing Benefits of Hydrotherapy

Introduction

*F*rom the time I was a child I've been interested in natural healing. My father would often say, "Your body knows how to heal itself...all you need to do is to give it a chance." This idea fascinated me, and helped to plant the seeds for what has become my life's work. The recent blossoming of interest in natural healing gives me immense pleasure. I think of the doctor who scoffed when I tried to discuss my interest in nutrition with him. "What you eat has virtually nothing to do with your health," he said. Although his comment seems preposterous now, our conversation took place merely twenty years ago. Another doctor at about the same time completely dismissed my theory that my lowered immunity was related to an extremely emotionally stressful time that I was going through.

Fortunately, I didn't listen to either "expert." I chose to trust the voice of my inner wisdom instead, and have found throughout the years that my best guide to health is my own body. I believe the same is true for you. After all, you have inhabited your body for all of your life—who can know it better than you? But understanding your body's messages takes practice, and your body's innate healing wisdom may be buried beneath layers of physical and emotional toxins. Many people are not even aware that they are suffering from toxic overload, and accept symptoms such as fatigue, headaches, depression, and digestive disturbances as normal. I can assure you that these symptoms are not normal, although you may have lots of fellow sufferers among your friends and acquaintances. Symptoms are the body's language of communication, and give you valuable feedback about what is working—and what isn't—in the way that you are taking care of yourself. When you clear out toxins, you provide your body and your mind with the opportunity for healing and rejuvenation.

Cleansing is an essential key for health. Our bodies are continually striving to maintain homeostasis, and the organs of detoxification are critical to this balancing act. The liver, kidneys, lungs, skin, lymphatic system, and intestinal tract are continually working to purify the body. They have a big job to do. We encounter many toxins in the course of a day, from environmental pollutants to the toxins produced by our own bodies as a by-product of normal metabolism. Even emotional stress creates physical toxins. While you can reduce the amount of toxins that you are exposed to, you can't avoid them entirely. But there are many things you can do to support your body's natural processes of detoxification. The 14-day program that I've outlined in this book is a gentle and effective plan for purifying your body and your mind and will help to reestablish the balance that creates optimal health.

My life-long interest in natural healing has enabled me to draw from a broad spectrum of healing modalities to create the purification program that I've designed for you. I began studying nutrition more than twenty-five years ago and have experimented with many different types of cleansing diets, from raw foods and fasting to a strict macrobiotic diet centered on brown rice, vegetables, and miso soup. I've practiced and taught yoga, meditation, and visualization for twenty years, and have studied the meditative martial arts of tai chi and chi kung. The intricate connection between the mind and the body has always fascinated me, and I earned a master's degree in clinical social work with an emphasis in behavioral medicine so that I could work with people to help them to restore their bodies and minds to health. My love of herbs infuses every aspect of my life, and I have relied on them as my primary form of medicine for more than two decades. All of these paths to healing have served me well, and have provided me with tools to help to keep my body in balance. I've discovered that when all organs and systems of the body are functioning in harmony, a state of radiant health naturally occurs.

Throughout the years I have experimented with a wide variety of cleansing programs, and I've found that the most effective program of purification is one that supports the organs of detoxification in a gentle and consistent way. I do not practice or recommend drastic methods of detoxification such as stringent fasts. Most people are unable to adhere to such a program even if they think it will benefit them, and harsh measures throw the body into a state of distress brought on by deprivation and the too quick release of toxins. In addition, rigid cleansing programs do nothing to teach you about really listening to your body, and do not bring about the types of long term changes that I believe are essential for true healing to occur.

I also know that for most of us, if something is pleasurable, we're more likely to continue doing it. The purification program that I recommend focuses on enjoyable, health-enhancing practices that you can incorporate into your daily life. During this 14-day herbal cleansing program, you'll nourish your body with delicious, healthful foods that promote cleansing and rejuvenation, and you'll learn how to use herbs to support your body's natural purification processes. You'll explore yoga and other ways of moving that stimulate energy flow and healing. You'll treat yourself to fragrant aromatherapy and herbal baths and massages, and learn breathing and relaxation techniques that will energize and refresh you. In addition, you'll explore the powerful connection between your mind and your body through journaling, visualization, and meditation. This is much more than just a fourteen-day program. What I share with you in this book is a way of life that offers you the opportunity to bring your mind, body, and spirit into harmony so that you can have all of your energy available for becoming all that you are meant to be. These natural methods of detoxification support the body's innate healing abilities, and help to open the subtle channels of energy flow. The cleansing program that I am offering to you is a way of reconnecting with your body's wisdom so that you can bring your body, mind, and spirit into alignment to achieve optimal health and well-being. I wish you joy in your journey!

Laurel Vukovic

PART ONE

CLEANSING: THE KEY TO OPTIMAL HEALTH

chapter one

How Cleansing Can Improve Your Health

Are you frequently fatigued, tense, or irritable? Is your digestion sluggish? Are you plagued by excess weight or cellulite? Do you suffer from joint pain, PMS, high cholesterol, allergies, or a diminished libido? What all of these problems, and the vast majority of degenerative diseases have in common, is the breakdown of your body's ability to maintain health. But regardless of the symptoms you may currently be experiencing, your body still strives to be healthy.

Every cell of your body is programmed to keep you in perfect health.

For example, at this very moment your liver is neutralizing toxins, your kidneys are purifying your blood, and your immune system is searching out and destroying invaders that threaten your wellbeing. Each system of your body works harmoniously in the intricate dance of life to keep you healthy.

Why Health Breakdowns Occur

If our bodies are so strongly programmed for health, why do we have health breakdowns? While there are a number of factors that lead to disease, many people overlook the most basic cause: *Disease occurs when our bodies are out of balance.* And although our bodies are programmed for health, it is possible to overwhelm your

3

body's ability to maintain balance. Think for a moment of the groggy way you waken in the morning after a late night out. Or the bone-tired exhaustion you feel after a long, stressful day at work. Or the sluggish, stuffed feeling you have after overindulging in a rich meal. These are all signals that you have thrown your body out of balance. For some people, these are occasional behaviors, and their bodies recover within a few hours or a couple of days. But for many people, these behaviors are a way of life, and become serious assaults on the body's ability to maintain equilibrium.

In today's complex world, many health assaults are accepted as normal. We are continually exposed to pollutants in our air, water, and soil. Eating meals on the run, fighting traffic, and financial and relationship worries keep levels of health-destroying stress hormones high. Habitually sitting for hours at desks, in cars, and in front of the television causes energy flow to stagnate. Circulation slows down, carbon dioxide builds up in the bloodstream, and liver, lymphatic, and intestinal function all become sluggish. The combination of stagnation and relentless assault by toxins impairs the normal functioning of the liver, lungs, large intestine, kidneys, skin, and lymphatic system, the organs reponsible for keeping the body clean and healthy. Your physical and emotional well-being are directly related to how efficiently your organs of detoxification are able to cleanse and purify your body.

We can never avoid toxins completely. Not only do we take in toxins through inhaling, ingesting, and coming into physical contact with them, but our bodies also produce toxins internally as a natural by-product of metabolic functioning. For example, normal intestinal bacteria create waste products that must be eliminated, and the digestion of proteins creates nitrogen wastes that are poisonous if not excreted by the kidneys. Simply defined, a *toxin* is any substance that irritates cells and interferes with the normal functioning of an organ. Toxicity occurs when excessive toxins are taken in, or when the body's normal pathways of detoxification are overloaded or blocked.

How Our Bodies Cleanse

Strong immune and eliminative functions are essential for the process of detoxification. The body handles toxins in two ways: By eliminating the offending substance, or by transforming the toxin into a less harmful substance. The major pathways of detoxification are the gastrointestinal system (including the liver, and colon), the respiratory system, the urinary system, the skin, and the lymphatic system. A good cleansing program supports organ function and the elimination of toxins. Helping your body cleanse in gentle, natural ways prevents the build-up of toxicity in your cells and organs and can dramatically improve your health.

PATHWAYS OF DETOXIFICATION

Liver

Large intestine

Kidneys

Lungs

Skin

Lymphatic system

Although our bodies evolved with the ability to neutralize and eliminate toxins, our organs were not designed to handle the levels of pollutants that we now encounter on a daily basis. The load of poisons we are exposed to overwhelms the organs of detoxification, and the resultant accumulation of toxins further impedes healthy organ functioning. The breakdown of the body's ability to neutralize and eliminate poisons lays the groundwork for many chronic and degenerative diseases. At the very least, even a low level of toxicity interferes with your ability to function optimally on all levels—physically, mentally, and emotionally.

For vibrant health and well-being, we need to support our organs of detoxification. We need to keep our energy flowing freely, and we need to reduce the amount of toxins we are exposed to. This includes not only external sources of toxins such as environmental pollutants, but internal toxins such as emotional stressors and patterns of negative thinking.

You can help to restore your body to radiant health
through simple practices of detoxification
and purification.

EVERYDAY TOXINS

Air pollution

Water pollution

Pesticides and herbicides

Food additives

Radiation

Prescription drugs

Recreational drugs

Synthetic bodycare products

Household and garden chemicals

Heavy metals

Mercury fillings

Refined foods

Caffeine

Alcohol

Tobacco

Overeating

Intestinal bacteria

Intestinal parasites

Lack of exercise

Emotional stressors

Insufficient sleep

Ancient Wisdom for Radiant Health

For centuries, wise healers in cultures around the world have known that vibrant well-being depends upon keeping the body balanced, and so they created methods of detoxification to clear the way for the body, mind, and spirit to function optimally. These purification practices are used to maintain health, prevent disease, promote mental clarity, and encourage spiritual enlightenment.

Some Native American tribes build ceremonial sweat lodges out of saplings covered with animal hides and gather around a pit filled with fiery-hot rocks. As the aromatic smoke of sweet grass, sage, and cedar fills the lodge, along with bursts of steam from ladles of water flung onto the smoldering rocks, the participants chant, sweat, and pray to purify and heal their bodies and spirits. In Chinese medicine, specific herbs are prescribed to eliminate conditions of excess that cause stagnation and disease, and the gentle martial arts forms of tai chi and chi kung are used to help unblock internal energy flow. The ancient Ayurvedic practices of India prescribe the regular use of elaborate cleansing and detoxification practices known as *pancha karma*. These techniques are employed to maintain health and promote longevity and include special foods and herbs, fragrant aromatherapy oil massages, and steam baths.

In all traditional cultures, rituals of cleansing and purification have been woven into the fabric of everyday life. What all of these detoxification practices have in common is the purification of the body through stimulating innate physical processes of detoxification. A natural clearing of the mind and a sense of spiritual clarity accompany this purification of the physical body. While these are powerful techniques of detoxification, they are also pleasant and often even richly sensual experiences that engender a sense of peace and unique well-being.

Creating Your Own Health Spa at Home

Many of these ancient purification practices have been adopted as healing and rejuvenation therapies at luxurious health and beauty spas. Saunas, steam baths, aromatherapy massages, herbal body wraps, seaweed baths, cleansing diets and juice fasts, and purifying herbal teas are a few of the detoxification practices offered at spas—for a thousand dollars or more per week. But you don't need to drain your savings account or go into debt to enjoy the benefits of a cleansing and rejuvenation program. In the comfort and privacy of your own home and for a fraction of the cost, you can recreate the finest spa treatments, tailored specifically to your needs and your schedule. For example, you can choose a one-day cleanse for a boost of energy and clarity, or embark on a two-week or longer deep cleansing purification program for healing or weight loss.

During the 14-day program outlined in this book, you'll provide your body with an opportunity to clear out toxins from your cells, and help your body come into balance so that rejuvenation can occur. Each day, you will enjoy nourishing foods that support optimal health. You'll spend one day on a more intensive deep cleansing fruit and vegetable fast to flush your cells with purifying nutrients. You'll include exercise in your daily routine to increase your circulation and energy flow, and you'll learn yoga postures to encourage healthy organ function and deep relaxation. You'll make herbal cleansing tonics to nurture and cleanse your body, and you'll enjoy a variety of luxurious herbal and aromatherapy bath and body treatments. To create a healthy mind in a healthy body, you'll learn techniques of breathing, meditation, and visualization that will help to purify your thinking and create a sense of deep calm. Woven together, these healing techniques create a powerful program of purification and rejuvenation.

You may find that you'll naturally begin to incorporate these pleasant practices into your daily health routines as you discover how these simple treatments dramatically improve your health and sense of well-being. Whether you choose a one-day or a one-month cleanse, you'll find that the time and energy you invest in a cleansing and rejuvenation program will richly reward you with improved physical, emotional, mental, and spiritual well-being.

Cleanse to Prevent Disease— From Colds to Cancer

One of the basic tenets of holistic medicine is the body's ability to self-regulate to maintain health. Your body is constantly striving to maintain *homeostasis*, or balance in the midst of constantly changing conditions. While you are busy going about your daily activities—working, running errands, managing a household, and meeting all of the other myriad demands on your time—your body is also busy internally with a variety of tasks that go on mostly beneath the level of your conscious awareness. Your digestive system is breaking down and assimilating nutrients and eliminating wastes. Your circulatory and respiratory systems are distributing nutrients and oxygen throughout your body. Your lymphatic system is cleansing your cells, your kidneys are purifying your bloodstream, and your skin is eliminating toxins through perspiration. Your immune system is constantly on patrol, fighting off invaders and scanning your body for unhealthy cells to destroy.

HOW YOU CAN HELP YOUR BODY CLEANSE

Cleansing diets

Juice fasting

Purifying herbs

Antioxidant supplements

Invigorating exercise

Yoga

Breathing exercises

Saunas

Steam baths

Aromatherapy baths

Massage

Emotional detoxification

Visualization

Meditation

Affirmations

Journal writing

Housecleaning for a Healthy Body

With such a heavy daily workload, it's essential to give your body a break to help it do some necessary housecleaning and repair work. Think of it like this: when your daily life responsibilities become too much of a burden, the first thing to slide is often the housework. Dust balls accumulate under the bed, spiders take over the corners, and odds and ends clutter the cabinets and drawers. Every so often, your home needs a thorough cleaning to restore order. It's the same with your body. When you provide your body with the opportunity to cleanse, the results can be remarkable. You'll experience an immediate lightness of body, mind, and spirit. Cleansing offers your body the opportunity to concentrate on healing and rejuvenation. There is no more potent, yet simple technique for improving your well-being on every level.

SYMPTOMS OF TOXICITY

Fatigue

Indigestion

Constipation

Bad breath

Acne

Skin rashes

Excess weight

Cellulite

Colds and flus

Sinus congestion

Joint pain

Muscle stiffness

Headaches

PMS

Depression

Anxiety

Insomnia

The Powerful Simplicity of Cleansing

You can incorporate the powerful concepts of detoxification into your daily life to help you achieve optimal health. While our systems are intricately designed to self-cleanse, providing your body with the assistance of purifying herbs, baths, massages, and other easy and pleasant rituals will help you to feel and look your best for your entire life.

While detoxification is at least as important as eating well, exercising, and taking supplements, it is often the missing component in a well-rounded and effective health program. I've seen many people add yet another dietary supplement to their already burgeoning medicine cabinets when they could achieve the benefits they are seeking through detoxification practices that support optimal organ functioning. I'm not against supplements—on the contrary, I use and recommend a variety of dietary supplements. But as Chinese and Ayurvedic healers discovered long ago, the body often needs to be cleansed before rejuvenating nutrients can be fully absorbed and utilized. Periodic deep cleansing offers the body an opportunity for self-renewal that no dietary supplement can provide.

How Excess Contributes to Disease

In our culture, we have a tendency to believe that more is better, and as a result, we are some of the most well-nourished people on the planet. The rich diet we have been privileged to eat—rich in proteins, fats, vitamins, and minerals—has caused us to grow bigger and taller and stronger with each generation. But the same diet also contributes to the formation and accumulation of excess; heart disease, clogged arteries, excess weight, blood sugar disturbances such as hypoglycemia and diabetes, chronic yeast infections, tumors and cancers are now understood to be caused primarily by our dietary and lifestyle habits. These are diseases of excess—essentially, diseases of toxicity.

I have witnessed many people undergo remarkable healings through adopting a cleansing program and a health-supportive lifestyle. I met Monika several years ago while I was teaching classes in natural foods cooking. She had been diagnosed with uterine cancer that had spread throughout her abdomen, and her doctors had told her that she had only six months to live. She radically changed her life, embracing a whole foods diet based on fresh vegetables and whole grains, practicing yoga and a form of Oriental self-massage daily, and taking walks in the fresh air. She used compresses and baths to increase circulation to her abdominal area, and practiced meditation and visualization. Instead of dying within six months, she became healthier than she had ever been, and to the astonishment of her doctors, her cancer disappeared.

Some people decide to take a detoxification approach because of serious illness. In many cases, it can help dramatically. Degenerative diseases are often the result of years of chronic low-level toxicity on a cellular level. By purifying your body, you are clearing the way for healing to occur. Our bodies are capable of miraculous changes, and are constantly striving to create a state of balance and optimal well-being. If you have a serious or chronic illness, please consult your health practitioner for help in designing an appropriate healing program.

DISEASES RELATED TO TOXICITY

Obesity

Allergies

Arthritis

Hypertension

Atherosclerosis

Cardiovascular disease

Cancer

Diabetes

Hypoglycemia

Menstrual disorders

Digestive disturbances

Skin disorders

Prostate problems

Cleansing: The Perfect Remedy for Eliminating Excess

The simplest remedy for the symptoms and diseases of excess is cleansing. Natural health practitioners believe that when the body is overloaded with toxins, disease occurs. The disease may be as commonplace as a cold or an allergy, or it can be as serious and life-threatening as the clogged arteries that lead to a heart attack or the damaged cells which give rise to cancer.

Many alternative healing programs for treating degenerative diseases are based on helping the body to cleanse. For example, physician Dean Ornish has proven that his program of dietary changes, exercise, and meditation reverses the clogged arteries associated with cardiovascular disease. His protocol is so successful that some insurance companies are willing to reimburse their clients who enroll in the program. From the insurance companies' point of view, Dr. Ornish's cleansing program has not only proven to be an effective treatment modality, but is also cheaper than a triple-bypass operation. And there's no question that a detoxification program is certainly a more pleasant option than surgery!

By incorporating detoxification practices into your life, you will help your body cleanse and achieve a state of optimal health. Why wait for a life-threatening illness to make changes in the way that you care for your body?

Remember, if you are suffering from a serious health problem, consult your doctor before undergoing a cleansing program. While detoxification can be an important aspect of helping to restore your body to health, a serious health breakdown requires a comprehensive healing program that addresses your individual needs.

Naturopathic physicians (N.D.s) are skilled in natural methods of healing, and many progressive M.D.s are beginning to see the wisdom of supporting the body's innate healing intelligence. Consult your health practitioner for advice in weaving together conventional medical treatments and natural healing modalities; there may be times when conventional medical treatments are necessary.

Whatever your current state of health, remember that your body has remarkable powers of rejuvenation. Ideally, include detoxification practices in your life as preventive medicine. Cleansing is an important key for helping your body to avoid the minor health breakdowns that lead to degenerative diseases.

Detoxify to Accelerate Healing

During any type of illness, our bodies increase their normal processes of detoxification. For example, when you come down with a cold or the flu, you naturally lose your appetite, because your body wants to focus attention on cleansing. You may run a fever, the body's natural internal mechanism for killing trouble-causing microorganisms. You may have copious mucus discharge and sneezing as your body attempts to expell the invaders. You can support your body in detoxifying and significantly cut short the duration of a cold or flu with cleansing therapies such as aromatherapy steams and mineral baths, purifying teas, and potent herbal remedies. In fact, by incorporating the principles of cleansing and detoxification into your daily life, you will be far less likely to fall prey to colds and flus.

My friend Maryanne used to come down with a cold or flu virus several times each year, and be sick for weeks at a time. When she asked for advice, I suggested that she eliminate refined foods, dairy products, and sugar, all of which weaken the immune system and create congestion. I also recommended that she eat plenty of garlic and ginger to help strengthen her immune system, and that she exercise daily, which has also been shown to enhance immune functioning. At the first sign of a cold or flu, I suggested that she take echinacea, a proven immune-enhancing tonic herb. The advice was simple, but effective. In the past two years, Maryanne has had one cold—and it only lasted a few days instead of for weeks.

HEALTH CHECK-UP SELF-TEST

Take this self-test now to determine your current level of health. Rate your response, and then total your responses for an indication of your general level of health. The higher your score, the more you will benefit from cleansing, and the greater your opportunity for health improvement. Be sure to take the test again at the end of your detoxification program to monitor your progress.

Use the following scoring: 1: Rarely 2: Sometimes 3: Often

SYMPTOMS OF TOXICITY

- ☐ I feel bloated or uncomfortable after eating.
- ☐ I have gas or indigestion after meals.
- ☐ I have hypoglycemia (low blood sugar).
- ☐ I am constipated.

- ☐ I have loose stools.
- ☐ My bowel movements contain undigested food.
- ☐ My bowel movements contain mucus.
- ☐ I have bad breath.
- ☐ My body odor is unpleasant.
- ☐ My urine is strong smelling or dark colored.
- ☐ I get urinary tract infections.
- ☐ I have sinusitis.
- ☐ I have nasal congestion.
- ☐ I have seasonal allergies.
- ☐ I have excess mucus in my lungs.
- ☐ My skin is prone to breaking out.
- ☐ I have clogged pores.
- ☐ My skin is excessively oily or dry.
- ☐ My skin is prone to rashes or eczema.
- ☐ My hair is excessively oily or dry.
- ☐ My hair is dull or has split ends.
- ☐ My nails split or break easily.
- ☐ I have bags or dark circles under my eyes.
- ☐ I am carrying excess weight on my body.
- ☐ I have cellulite.
- ☐ My joints ache or are stiff.
- ☐ My muscles ache or are sore.
- ☐ I feel fatigued.
- ☐ I am irritable, depressed, or anxious.
- ☐ My thinking is foggy or unclear.
- ☐ I experience a slump in energy in the afternoon.
- ☐ I get headaches.
- ☐ I have difficulty falling asleep at night.
- ☐ I wake up during the night.
- ☐ I have difficulty getting up in the morning.
- ☐ I get out of breath easily.
- ☐ I get colds and flus.
- ☐ When I get sick, it takes me a long time to recover.

☐ When I get cut, it takes a long time to heal.

☐ I look older than my age.

☐ My sexual vitality is less than I would like.

For Women:

☐ I have PMS symptoms such as bloating and irritability.

☐ My menstrual cycles are irregular.

☐ I get menstrual cramps.

☐ My menstrual flow is excessively heavy.

☐ I get vaginal yeast infections.

For Men:

☐ I have prostatitis.

☐ I have an enlarged prostate gland.

SIGNS OF HEALTH AND VITALITY

For this section, use the following scoring:

1: Often 2: Sometimes 3: Rarely

☐ I digest my food easily.

☐ My stomach feels comfortable after eating.

☐ I have one or more bowel movements daily.

☐ My bowel movements are well-formed and odorless.

☐ My breath smells sweet.

☐ My body odor is pleasant.

☐ My urine is light colored.

☐ I urinate every couple of hours.

☐ My skin is smooth and blemish free.

☐ My skin has a healthy, glowing look.

☐ My hair is shiny.

☐ My nails are strong.

☐ My eyes are bright and clear.

☐ My weight is ideal for my body.

☐ My body is flexible.

☐ I have good muscle tone.

☐ I have good endurance.

☐ I have plenty of energy for whatever I want to do.

☐ My energy remains steady throughout the day.

☐ My thinking is clear.

☐ I go to sleep within minutes after going to bed.

☐ I sleep through the night without waking.

☐ I awake refreshed.

☐ I sleep between 6 and 10 hours a night.

☐ I am generally happy.

☐ My emotions are stable.

☐ I rarely get sick.

☐ When I do get sick, I recover quickly.

☐ If I get cut, I heal quickly.

☐ I look younger than my age.

☐ I have plenty of sexual vitality.

For women only:

☐ My menstrual cycles are regular and pain free.

For men only:

☐ My prostate gland is healthy.

chapter two

The Physical, Mental, and Emotional Benefits of Cleansing

Cleanse to Look Your Best

For many people, making changes that will help them to look better is more highly motivating than making changes that will help them to live longer. It doesn't really matter if your primary motivation is to improve your health or to improve your appearance. When you begin to incorporate practices of purification into your life, you will reap the benefits of both, because true beauty is a state of radiant health.

To a great extent, your external appearance is a direct reflection of your internal state of well-being. When your organs of detoxification are functioning well, your cells and tissues are cleansed and rejuvenated, and you begin to glow with health. Excess pounds drop away as your metabolism begins to work more efficiently. Eyes and skin become clear as toxins are released, and hair and nails become strong and healthy as nutrients are better absorbed. On a more subtle level, inner health manifests externally as a radiance that is magnetically attractive. When you help your body to come into a state of balance, your unique beauty shines!

Be sure to treat yourself to spa beauty treatments, not only while you're cleansing, but on a regular basis. Facials and bodycare treatments are nurturing and help to bring forth your beauty. See

Chapter 15 for a wealth of suggestions and recipes for pampering yourself. Whatever your reasons for undertaking a cleansing program, you can be certain that you will look and feel better, and be healthier in body, mind, and spirit. Enjoy all of the benefits of this wonderful commitment that you are making to your well-being!

Detoxify to Achieve Your Ideal Weight

Overweight is a form of excess, and is often a sign that the body is not metabolizing food properly. However, it's important to realize that the human form comes in a variety of beautiful shapes and sizes, and if we are to be truly healthy, we need to love and accept the natural shape of our bodies. Don't judge your body by the scale or by a weight chart. Instead, look at your body carefully and lovingly and notice without criticism if you are carrying excess weight that you would like to release. Focus on cultivating an inner sense of how you would like to feel in your body independent of the number on a scale.

If you are nourishing your body with healthy foods, eating in accordance with your true physical hunger, and providing your body with the exercise it craves to feel energetic and relaxed, you will effortlessly gravitate toward your ideal natural weight. If you do want to lighten up a bit, a detoxification program is a wonderful way to release excess. Most people find that extra pounds melt away when they adopt the principles of cleansing and detoxification. Joanne, one of my students, had struggled with trying to lose twenty pounds for years. She tried every diet imaginable, but inevitably, the pounds she so painfully lost would creep back on within a few months. After taking one of my classes, she decided to try a gentle purification program, and lost a few pounds within a couple of weeks. More importantly, her digestion improved, she had more energy for exercise, and she began for the first time to make friends with her body. She nourished her body with the finest fresh, organic foods, found ways of exercising that felt good, and indulged in aromatherapy baths, saunas, and massages. As she integrated the principles of cleansing into her daily life, she easily lost all of the excess weight she had been carrying without any feelings of deprivation.

I have seen many people successfully lose weight when they focus on supporting their bodies' innate desire for perfect health. Purification practices bring the body into balance, and offer a natural method of weight control that facilitates optimal well-being. A cleansing diet, detoxifying herbs, and supplements that improve digestion and elimination help the body to process foods more efficiently. Purifying exercises, cleansing breathing techniques, massage, and visualization practices encourage a harmonious balance of body, mind, and spirit that naturally results in the achievement of the perfect weight and shape for your body. The self-nurturing practices of cleansing provide an opportunity for you to get in touch with your body and heighten your awareness of your internal processes.

If you suffer from an eating disorder such as anorexia or bulimia, do not undergo a cleansing or detoxification program without the supervision of a health practitioner.

How Toxins Cause Aging

A detoxification program offers your body an opportunity for renewal on a cellular level. Each day, your organs are faced with the job of general systems maintenance. In addition, your body must keep up with the never-ending task of neutralizing toxins, preventing damage to cells, and repairing any damage that has occurred. When you embark on a cleansing program, you reduce the load of toxins that your body has to deal with and you provide support for your organs in their detoxification work. This frees up increased energy for the repair work that rejuvenates your cells and organs.

Much of what we think of and accept as part of the normal aging process is in fact caused by the build-up of toxins in our cells and tissues. Under a heavy or unrelenting load of toxins, the body struggles just to maintain the daily functioning of vital body processes. Have you ever wondered why your digestion is just not what it used to be, why your sleep is fitful, or why your supply of energy can barely get you through the day? Perhaps you look in the mirror and see dull, blotchy skin, lines of tiredness, and eyes that are less than sparkling. Slumped posture, slack muscles, and various aches and pains are other signs of aging that we all too often accept as normal.

Reverse the Signs of Aging Through Cleansing

In even the first few hours of a cleansing program, you will notice an immediate feeling of well-being as your body turns its attention to rejuvenation. Instead of laboring under a heavy load of toxic build-up, your body will be free to repair and renew cells. As a result, your energy will increase and you'll experience a renewed zest for living. Your sleep will be more peaceful and you'll awaken refreshed, with a clear mind. Your digestion will improve, as will your elimination. You'll notice that your eyes are clear when you look into the mirror, and your skin will become soft and smooth. Your posture will improve as you become more aware of your body, and you'll feel a delightful lightness of your body, mind, and spirit.

Unlike some detoxification programs that require strict fasts or other stringent measures, I believe that the healthiest program of detoxification is one that makes you feel great while you're doing it. Cultivate the practice of listening to your body's internal messages. If what you are doing makes you feel healthy, joyful, energetic, loving, and creative, then you're on the right track. If you feel cranky, angry, depressed, and tired, then it's time to reevaluate. There are many paths to health. Be gentle with yourself and choose a path that feels good to you.

THE PHYSICAL BENEFITS OF CLEANSING

Improved health

Increased energy

Better digestion

Restful sleep

Smooth skin

Loss of excess weight

Enhanced flexibility

The Mental and Emotional Benefits of Cleansing

While most cleansing programs focus on the physical benefits of detoxification, there are many emotional and mental benefits that you will experience as well. Our bodies, minds, and spirits are intricately interwoven, and everything we do affects each part of our being.

Detoxify for Bright and Creative Mental Energy

Detoxification sharpens your mental focus, helping you to concentrate more fully on whatever task is in front of you. If you live a typically modern lifestyle, you may rarely be functioning at your optimal level of bright and creative mental energy. Recall, for instance, of how you feel after eating a heavy lunch. You probably find it difficult to concentrate, and your thinking becomes fuzzy around the edges. In addition, if you've been sitting all day, your energy flow is stagnant. At this point, many people find they have an almost overwhelming desire to take a nap. That's why afternoon coffee breaks are taken for granted in many workplaces—caffeine and sugar provide an unnatural surge of energy to propel employees through the rest of the day. When you adopt a nontoxic lifestyle that includes cleansing practices, your mental focus will sharpen and your creative impulses will flow freely and steadily, without the need for artificial and harmful stimulants.

Improve Your Memory Through Cleansing

Cleansing can also help to improve your memory. Although we resign ourselves to memory loss as another inevitable aspect of aging, memory impairment is frequently caused by clogged arteries leading to the brain. The brain requires nutrients and oxygen to function, and if the supply is diminished because of decreased blood flow through narrowed arteries, the result is often a decrease in mental functioning, including memory recall. The same overload of toxins that causes fuzzy thinking also contributes to memory loss. By incorporating techniques of detoxification, particularly through diet, exercise, cleansing herbs and other supplements, brain function can often be improved. Many people report an almost immediate increase in clarity of thinking, including sharper memory, when they begin a program of cleansing.

My friend Jon complained that he was having difficulty staying focused in his work, and felt that his memory was slipping. Sometimes he even blanked out on the names of close friends. Jon often skipped lunch, and to stay alert, he drank pots of coffee, and then had a large meal and a couple of drinks when he finally arrived home in the evening. I explained to him that he was suffering from symptoms of toxicity, and that caffeine and alcohol are two of the primary stressors on the liver and other organs of detoxification. I suggested that he eliminate caffeine and alcohol and eat regular meals throughout the day, with plenty of fresh vegetables and fruits to help his body cleanse. I also recommended that he drink a liver-cleansing herbal tea for a couple of weeks, along with taking milk thistle extract for liver rejuvenation, and that he take time every day for a brisk walk to get some fresh air and exercise to improve the circulation to his brain. Jon suffered from caffeine withdrawal for a few days, but afterward, reported feeling more energy and sharper thinking than he had experienced in years.

Cleanse to Relieve Depression and Anxiety

Undertaking a purifying cleanse can have profound positive effects on your mental state. Even choosing to begin a program of detoxification is empowering. By making a conscious decision to improve your well-being and taking definite steps in the direction of health, you are affirming to yourself that you are important.

Negative emotional states are commonplace in our society, with depression and anxiety perhaps the most widespread complaints. While it is normal to experience a wide range of emotions, a chronic or frequent state of depression or anxiety diminishes the life force and severely disrupts all aspects of a person's life. Depression and anxiety are often rooted in deeply held beliefs, and a person who suffers from these painful emotions can benefit greatly from the help of a good therapist.

At the same time, a program of purification can help to bring the body into balance, exerting a calming and centering influence on the emotions. In Chinese medicine, the liver is believed to rule emotions such as depression and anxiety. Specific cleansing foods and herbs as well as lifestyle changes can help to detoxify and harmonize the liver and restore a healthy and balanced perspective to life and the challenges it brings.

Stabilize Mood Swings Through Detoxification

Some people experience depression and anxiety only intermittently. For example, many women suffer from premenstrual or menopausal depression or anxiety. Many times, these mood shifts are more related to hormonal fluctuations than to any deeply rooted psychological disturbances. However, any issues that torment you premenstrually or during menopause are likely to be real concerns in your life that are brought to your awareness and intensified by the hormonal fluctuations. In other words, pay attention to what your emotions are telling you! Unresolved emotions have toxic effects on your body, mind, and spirit. While you are honoring your emotional process, a program of detoxification can help to smooth out hormonal imbalances.

Celeste, one of my students, was 43 and beginning to go through the hormonal changes that precede menopause. She was alternately depressed and irritable, and confided that at times she felt that she was losing her mind. She began a cleansing program, paying close attention to her diet and taking herbs specifically chosen to help detoxify her liver. She also began attending yoga classes twice a week and treated herself to a massage a couple of times a month. The changes Celeste made in her life helped her body to more easily detoxify the problem-causing hormones, and she began feeling more energetic, calm, and centered within a few weeks. By adopting simple cleansing practices, Celeste gave herself the gift of self-nurturing, which had profound effects on her emotional and physical well-being.

Cleanse and Clear Negative Thought Patterns

The mind and body are inextricably intertwined, and undertaking a detoxification program will help to cleanse not only your body, but your mind as well. Negative thought patterns are a subtle and often unconscious form of toxicity.

Begin to bring your thought patterns into conscious awareness by paying attention to your thoughts and to the effects that they have on your mental and physical well-being. If your thoughts are primarily negative, they will have a destructive effect on your body. Have you ever noticed that you are more likely to become sick when you feel stressed or unhappy? Negative emotions suppress the immune system, and have been shown to be a factor in the development of both acute and chronic diseases.

Mary, one of my students, suffered from chronic digestive distress with symptoms of severe intestinal cramps and alternating diarrhea and constipation. Her doctor diagnosed her as having colitis, and prescribed medication which only partially controlled the symptoms. Mary went on a cleansing program, which provided only moderate relief. Because of the strong link between colitis and emotions, I suggested that Mary consider psychotherapy. As she began to uncover buried feelings, Mary recognized that unexpressed emotions had been literally eating away at her. She learned to identify and express her feelings in a healthy way, and as a result, is symptom free.

If your thoughts are primarily positive, you will feel a natural joy that will enhance the health of every cell of your being. When you embark on a cleansing program, you are embracing your power to positively affect your health, and you are automatically supporting and affirming the natural healing abilities of your body.

MENTAL-EMOTIONAL BENEFITS OF CLEANSING

Memory improvement

Enhanced creativity

Sharper mental focus

Stable moods

Increased joy

Sense of well-being

Your Body's Natural Healing Intelligence

We are blessed with incredible powers of self-renewal. Because healing occurs beneath the level of our conscious awareness, we may take it for granted. Consider for a moment the ease with which your body repairs a minor cut, and fully acknowledge that your body has the ability to heal virtually any disease or injury that you might encounter. Cultivating awareness of this ability can stimulate healing. At the same time that we express gratitude and confidence in the miracle of self-renewal, we sometimes need to get out of the way so that the body can heal. I believe that our bodies give us messages that guide us to vibrant health. But all too often, we are so accustomed to high levels of stressful behavior that we cannot hear the messages.

Listening to Your Body

Cleansing is an effective means for getting out of the way and allowing the body's natural healing wisdom to prevail. Your body's signals are much easier to hear when you don't override its messages with too much food, not enough sleep or rest, and stressors such as sugar, alcohol, and caffeine. It might take some experimentation, especially if you've been living a typically modern lifestyle and have become somewhat disconnected from your body. Don't be discouraged—begin where you are, without any self-judgments. Remember that creating optimal health is a journey. If you set out with the intention of enjoying the process, you won't be disappointed.

Recognize that you have the choice in every moment of your life to be moving either toward vibrant health or disease.

Don't wait until you are sick to begin listening to your body. Cultivate the willingness to hear what your body is telling you now. Are you hungry, or thirsty? What would satisfy your hunger or thirst now? Are you attuned to your body's signals of having eaten enough? Do you honor your body's need to move, and do you rest when you are tired? Do you stretch when you feel a tense muscle, and take a few deep breaths when you feel anxious or rushed? Get into the habit of checking in with yourself, and practice meeting your needs in the moment. Cultivating an attitude of awareness along with regular practices of detoxification will help you to become attuned to your body's wisdom.

LISTENING TO YOUR BODY

Take just a moment to tune in to your body,
and ask yourself the following questions:

Am I thirsty?

Am I hungry?

Do I need to stretch?

Do I need to rest?

Do I need to exercise?

Do I need to breathe?

Do I need some quiet time?

Do I need to talk with a friend?

Do I need a hug?

What do I need to come into balance now?

The Benefits of Paying Attention

A healthful lifestyle includes eating a cleansing, nourishing diet of fresh, seasonal foods; exercising to keep your energy flowing and your organs functioning optimally; sufficient rest for renewal and healing; and focusing your thoughts in a positive direction. Paying exquisite attention to your body will help you to stay in balance. The benefits are immediate—you'll feel better physically, emotionally, mentally, and spiritually.

By being aware of the first subtle signals of imbalance, you can take action and avert a more serious illness. For example, I've learned that the first sign my body gives me of an impending cold or flu is a subtle feeling of fatigue and an almost imperceptible scratchy sensation at the back of my throat. If I pay attention immediately and take steps to help my body fight the virus, I can avoid becoming sick. I make a pot of soup rich with immune-boosting herbs, drink cleansing herbal teas, take a hot bath with purifying essential oils, and get plenty of rest. These cleansing treatments are pleasant and self-nurturing, and I almost always wake up the next morning without any sign of illness.

The Best Form of Health Insurance

Detoxification is one of the most powerful tools you have available for preventing disease and creating radiant health. As you experiment with the various techniques of cleansing and detoxification, you will discover an energizing, uplifting, and healing experience awaits you. You may choose, as I and many of my students do, to incorporate these simple practices into your daily life. Think of detoxification as a form of health insurance, for everything you do to help your body in its natural process of purification will reward you with increased vitality and zest for life.

chapter three

14-Day Herbal Cleansing and Rejuvenation Program

*T*he following program takes you through 14 days of purifying, healing, and rejuvenating activities. Each day, you will eat a healthful diet centered around foods that support your body's natural cleansing processes. For a more intensive cleansing experience, you'll spend the seventh day fasting on fresh vegetable and fruit juices or simple vegetable soups. You'll cultivate the habit of daily exercise, and learn energizing stretches, rejuvenating yoga postures, and purifying breathing exercises. You'll learn to use the power of your mind to enhance your cleansing experience as you practice deep relaxation, journal writing, meditation, and visualization. You'll prepare and drink purifying herbal teas and other beverages each day, and you'll enjoy the benefits of spa treatments in your own home with herbal and aromatherapy baths, massages, and luxurious bodycare treatments.

In only two weeks, you can refresh your body, mind, and spirit and enjoy significant changes in your mental and physical health. This purification program is infinitely flexible; feel free to make any adjustments you wish to suit your needs and desires. For the greatest long-term benefits, incorporate these wonderful health-supportive activities into your daily life. Enjoy your journey to vibrant well-being!

Day 1

Morning Cleansing Activities:

- Upon arising, drink a glass of pure water with a squeeze of fresh lemon or lime juice
- Prepare Herbal Purifying Tea #1 (p. 134) and drink 3 cups throughout the day between meals

Diet:

- Eliminate dietary stressors such as caffeine and alcohol, processed foods, white flour, sugar, saturated and polyunsaturated fats, dairy products, and red meat
- Follow Health Enhancing Diet (p. 154)
- Take Herbal Bitters Tonic (p. 126) before meals if desired to improve digestion

Exercise:

- Take a 15-minute walk in the morning, afternoon, or evening

Evening Cleansing Activities:

- Enjoy a 20-minute Aromatherapy Bath (p. 207)
- Begin a journal to enhance your detoxification experience (p. 245)
- Go to bed before 10:00 P.M.

Day 2

Morning Cleansing Activities:

- Upon arising, drink a glass of pure water with a squeeze of fresh lemon or lime juice
- Take Intestinal Cleansing Beverage (p. 81)
- Prepare Herbal Purifying Tea #2 (p. 134) and drink 3 cups throughout the day between meals
- Finish your morning shower with a cold water rinse to stimulate lymphatic flow

Diet:

- Ꙩ Follow Health Enhancing Diet (p. 154)
- Ꙩ Take Herbal Bitters Tonic (p. 126) before meals if desired to improve digestion

Exercise:

- Ꙩ Take a 15-minute walk in the morning, afternoon, or evening
- Ꙩ Practice 15 minutes of Energizing Stretches (p. 188) whenever you choose

Evening Cleansing Activities:

- Ꙩ Practice Diaphragmatic Breathing (p. 232) just before bed
- Ꙩ Journal Writing (p. 245)
- Ꙩ Go to bed before 10:00 P.M.

Day 3

Morning Cleansing Activities:

- Ꙩ Upon arising, drink a glass of pure water with a squeeze of fresh lemon or lime juice
- Ꙩ Take Intestinal Cleansing Beverage (p. 81)
- Ꙩ Prepare Herbal Purifying Tea #1 (p. 134) and drink 3 cups throughout the day between meals
- Ꙩ Perform Dry Brush Massage (p. 236) before showering, and finish your shower with a cold rinse

Diet:

- Ꙩ Follow Health Enhancing Diet (p. 154)
- Ꙩ Take Herbal Bitters Tonic (p. 126) before meals if desired to improve digestion

Exercise:

- Ꙩ Take a 20-minute walk in the morning, afternoon, or evening
- Ꙩ Practice 15 minutes of Energizing Stretches (p. 188) whenever you choose

Evening Cleansing Activities:

- ⌒ Practice Meditation on the Breath (p. 251)
- ⌒ Enjoy Sea and Earth Mineral Bath (p. 208) before bed
- ⌒ Journal Writing (p. 245)
- ⌒ Go to bed before 10:00 P.M.

Day 4

Morning Cleansing Activities:

- ⌒ Upon arising, drink a glass of pure water with a squeeze of fresh lemon or lime juice
- ⌒ Perform Hot Towel Scrub (p. 236) to stimulate lymphatic flow
- ⌒ Practice Vitality Enhancing Breath (p. 234)
- ⌒ Take Intestinal Cleansing Beverage (p. 81)
- ⌒ Prepare Herbal Purifying Tea #2 (p. 134) and drink 3 cups throughout the day between meals

Diet:

- ⌒ Follow Health Enhancing Diet (p. 154)
- ⌒ Take Herbal Bitters Tonic (p. 126) before meals if desired to improve digestion

Exercise:

- ⌒ Take a 20-minute walk in the morning, afternoon, or evening
- ⌒ Practice 20 minutes of Rejuvenating Yoga Postures whenever you choose

Evening Cleansing Activities:

- ⌒ Enjoy a relaxing Aromatherapy massage (p. 240) with your partner or a friend, or perform Lymph-Cleansing Massage (p. 237)
- ⌒ Journal Writing (p. 245)
- ⌒ Go to bed before 10:00 P.M.

Day 5

Morning Cleansing Activities:

- Upon arising, drink a glass of pure water with a squeeze of fresh lemon or lime juice
- Practice Recharge Breath (p. 233)
- Take Intestinal Cleansing Beverage (p. 81)
- Prepare Herbal Purifying Tea #1 (p. 134) and drink 3 cups throughout the day between meals

Diet:

- Follow Health Enhancing Diet (p. 154)
- Take Herbal Bitters Tonic (p. 126) before meals if desired to improve digestion

Exercise:

- Take a 25-minute walk in the morning, afternoon, or evening
- Practice 15 minutes of Energizing Stretches whenever you choose

Evening Cleansing Activities:

- Enjoy Herbal Deep Detoxifying Bath (p. 215) before bed
- Drink a cup of Purifying and Relaxing Herbal Tea (p. 215) while in the bath
- Journal Writing (p. 245)
- Practice Progressive Relaxation exercise (p. 247) before sleeping
- Go to bed before 10:00 P.M.

Day 6

Morning Cleansing Activities:

- Upon arising, drink a glass of Purifying Aloe Drink (p. 128)
- Practice Deep Cleansing Breath (p. 234)

🌀 Prepare Herbal Purifying Tea #2 and drink 3 cups throughout the day between meals

🌀 Take Intestinal Cleansing Beverage (p. 81)

Diet:

🌀 *Breakfast:*
Fresh fruit or Gingered Fruit Compote (p. 182)

🌀 *Lunch:*
2-3 servings lightly cooked and raw vegetables
3-4 ounces lean protein: fish, poultry, tofu, etc.
Season with olive oil, lemon, herbs, and sea salt

🌀 *Dinner:*
2-3 servings lightly cooked and raw vegetables
1-2 servings complex carbohydrates: brown rice, potatoes, corn, etc.
Season with olive oil, lemon, herbs, and sea salt

🌀 *Snacks:*
Fresh fruit, raw vegetables, fresh vegetable juices

Exercise:

🌀 Take a 30-minute walk in the morning, afternoon, or evening

🌀 Practice 20 minutes of Rejuvenating Yoga Postures (p. 191) whenever you choose

Evening Cleansing Activities:

🌀 Enjoy Lymph Stimulating Foot Bath (p. 216)

🌀 Practice Meditation on a Mantra (p. 251)

🌀 Apply Scalp Conditioning Treatment (p. 225) and leave on overnight

🌀 Drink Gentle Laxative Tea (p. 130) before bed

🌀 Journal Writing (p. 245)

🌀 Go to bed before 10:00 P.M.

Day 7

Morning Cleansing Activities:

- Upon arising, practice Abdominal Cleansing Breath (p. 235)
- Practice 10 minutes of Energizing Stretches (p. 188)
- Drink a glass of Purifying Aloe Drink (p. 128)
- Prepare Herbal Purifying Tea #1 (p. 134) and drink 3 cups throughout the day between meals
- Take Intestinal Cleansing Beverage (p. 81)
- Apply Body Purifying Scrub (p. 211) during morning shower and finish with a cold water rinse

Diet:

- Purifying Fast Day: (see p. 155 for guidelines)
  Choose from:
  Fresh vegetable and fruit juices (p. 157)
  Vegetable broth and soups (p. 164)
  Steamed vegetables
- Have juice, soup, and/or vegetables every 2-3 hours
- Drink 3 cups of Herbal Purifying Tea throughout the day
- Drink hot lemon water as desired throughout the day

Exercise:

- Take a gentle 30-minute walk in the morning, afternoon, or evening
- Practice 20 minutes of Rejuvenating Yoga Postures (p. 191) whenever you choose

Afternoon and Evening Cleansing Activities:

- Practice Alternate Nostril Breathing (p. 234)
- Practice Candle Gazing Meditation (p. 252)
- Enjoy Relaxing Herbal Detoxifying Soak (p. 214)
- Apply Strawberry Exfoliating Mask (p. 223) while in the tub
- Drink Gentle Laxative Tea (p. 130) before bed

🌱 Journal Writing (p. 245)
🌱 Go to bed before 10:00 P.M.

Day 8

Morning Cleansing Activities:

🌱 Perform Abdominal Massage (p. 235)
🌱 Drink a glass of Purifying Aloe Drink (p. 128)
🌱 Practice 10 minutes of Energizing Stretches (p. 188)
🌱 Prepare Herbal Purifying Tea #2 and drink 3 cups throughout the day between meals
🌱 Take Intestinal Cleansing Beverage (p. 81)
🌱 Finish your morning shower with a cold water rinse to stimulate lymphatic flow

Diet:

🌱 *Breakfast:*
Fresh fruit or Gingered Fruit Compote (p. 182)
🌱 *Lunch:*
2-3 servings lightly cooked and raw vegetables
1-2 servings complex carbohydrates: brown rice, potatoes, corn, etc.
Season with olive oil, lemon, herbs, and sea salt
🌱 *Dinner:*
2-3 servings lightly cooked and raw vegetables
3-4 ounces lean protein: fish, poultry, tofu, etc.
Season with olive oil, lemon, herbs, and sea salt
🌱 *Snacks:*
Fresh fruit, raw vegetables, vegetable juices

Exercise:

🌱 Take a 30-minute walk in the morning, afternoon, or evening
🌱 Practice 20 minutes of Rejuvenating Yoga postures (p. 191) whenever you choose

Evening Cleansing Activities:

- Enjoy a sauna or Epsom Salts Detoxifying Bath (p. 207)
- Perform Lymph-Cleansing Massage (p. 237) or Cellulite Massage (p. 238) while in the sauna or bath
- Journal Writing (p. 245)
- Go to bed before 10:00 P.M.

Day 9

Morning Cleansing Activities:

- Upon arising, drink a glass of Purifying Aloe Drink (p. 128)
- Practice 10 minutes of Energizing Stretches (p. 188)
- Prepare Herbal Purifying Tea #1 (p. 134) and drink 3 cups throughout the day between meals
- Take Intestinal Cleansing Beverage (p. 81)
- Perform Dry Brush Massage (p. 236) before morning shower

Diet:

- Follow Health Enhancing Diet (p. 154)
- Take Herbal Bitters Tonic (p. 126) before meals if desired to improve digestion

Exercise:

- Take a 30-minute walk in the morning, afternoon, or evening
- Practice 20 minutes of Rejuvenating Yoga Postures (p. 191) whenever you choose

Evening Cleansing Activities:

- Practice Healing Visualization (p. 252)
- Journal Writing (p. 245)
- Go to bed before 10:00 P.M.

Day 10

Morning Cleansing Activities:

- Upon arising, drink a glass of Purifying Aloe Drink (p. 128)
- Practice Deep Cleansing Breath (p. 234)
- Practice 10 minutes of Energizing Stretches (p. 188)
- Prepare Herbal Purifying Tea #2 (p. 134) and drink 3 cups through-out the day between meals
- Take Intestinal Cleansing Beverage (p. 81)
- Finish morning shower with a cold water rinse to stimulate lymphatic flow

Diet:

- Follow Health Enhancing Diet (p. 154)
- Take Herbal Bitters Tonic (p. 126) before meals if desired to improve digestion

Exercise:

- Take a 30-minute walk in the morning, afternoon, or evening
- Practice 20 minutes of Rejuvenating Yoga Postures whenever you choose

Evening Cleansing Activities:

- Enjoy Eucalyptus-Seaweed Detoxifying Soak (p. 209)
- Practice Meditation on the Breath (p. 251)
- Journal Writing (p. 245)
- Go to bed before 10:00 P.M.

Day 11

Morning Cleansing Activities:

- Upon arising, drink a glass of Purifying Aloe Drink (p. 128)

- Practice Complete Breath (p. 233)
- Prepare Herbal Purifying Tea #2 (p. 134) and drink 3 cups throughout the day between meals
- Take Intestinal Cleansing Beverage (p. 81)
- Finish morning shower with a cold water rinse to stimulate lymphatic flow

Diet:

- Follow Health Enhancing Diet (p. 154)
- Take Herbal Bitters (p. 126) before meals if desired to improve digestion

Exercise:

- Take a 30-minute walk in the morning, afternoon, or evening
- Practice 20 minutes of Rejuvenating Yoga Postures (p. 191) whenever you choose

Evening Cleansing Activities:

- Practice Healing Visualization (p. 252)
- Perform Hot Towel Scrub before bed (p. 236)
- Journal Writing (p. 245)
- Go to bed before 10:00 P.M.

Day 12

Morning Cleansing Activities:

- Upon arising, drink a glass of Purifying Aloe Drink (p. 128)
- Practice 10 minutes of Energizing Stretches (p. 188)
- Prepare Herbal Purifying Tea #1 and drink 3 cups throughout the day between meals
- Take Intestinal Cleansing Beverage (p. 81)
- Finish morning shower with a cold water rinse to stimulate lymphatic flow

Diet:

- ᔣ Follow Health Enhancing Diet (p. 154)
- ᔣ Take Herbal Bitters Tonic (p. 126) before meals if desired to improve digestion

Exercise:

- ᔣ Take a 30-minute walk in the morning, afternoon, or evening
- ᔣ Practice 20 minutes of Rejuvenating Yoga Postures whenever you choose

Evening Cleansing Activities:

- ᔣ Enjoy Relaxing Herbal Detoxifying Soak (p. 214)
- ᔣ Apply Honey-Lavender Mask (p. 223) while in the bath
- ᔣ Journal Writing (p. 245)
- ᔣ Go to bed before 10:00 P.M.

Day 13

Morning Cleansing Activities:

- ᔣ Upon arising, drink a glass of pure water with a squeeze of fresh lemon or lime juice
- ᔣ Prepare Herbal Purifying Tea #2 (p. 134) and drink 3 cups throughout the day between meals
- ᔣ Practice Diaphragmatic Breathing (p. 232)
- ᔣ Take Intestinal Cleansing Beverage (p. 81)
- ᔣ Use Skin Renewing All-Over Body Exfoliant (p. 212) in shower and finish with a cold water rinse

Diet:

- ᔣ Follow Health Enhancing Diet (p. 154)
- ᔣ Take Herbal Bitters Tonic (p. 126) before meals if desired to improve digestion

Exercise:

- Take a 30-minute walk in the morning, afternoon, or evening
- Practice 20 minutes of Rejuvenating Yoga Postures (p. 191) whenever you choose

Evening Cleansing Activities:

- Enjoy a relaxing Aromatherapy Massage (p. 240) with your partner or a friend, or a Lymph Cleansing Massage (p. 237)
- Journal Writing (p. 245)
- Go to bed before 10:00 P.M.

Day 14

Morning Cleansing Activities:

- Upon arising, drink a glass of pure water with a squeeze of fresh lemon or lime juice
- Practice Vitality Enhancing Breath (p. 234)
- Practice 10 minutes of Energizing Stretches (p. 188)
- Prepare Herbal Purifying Tea #1 (p. 134) and drink 3 cups throughout the day between meals
- Take Intestinal Cleansing Beverage (p. 81)

Diet:

- Follow Health Enhancing Diet (p. 154)
- Take Herbal Bitters Tonic (p. 126) before meals if desired to improve digestion

Exercise:

- Take a 30-minute walk in the morning, afternoon, or evening
- Practice 20 minutes of Rejuvenating Yoga Postures whenever you choose

Afternoon and Evening Cleansing Activities:

⌣ Treat yourself to a full Spa Day (p. 229), including a complete facial, conditioning hair treatment, pedicure, and manicure

⌣ Enjoy Relaxation with Music (p. 249)

⌣ Journal Writing (p. 245)

⌣ Go to bed before 10:00 P.M.

chapter four

Creating
a Healthful Lifestyle

Reducing Your Exposure to Toxins

When you initiate a program of cleansing and detoxification, begin by considering the ways that you can reduce the number of toxins that you encounter on a daily basis. Our bodies were not designed to cope with large amounts of pollutants, or to metabolize or eliminate synthetic chemicals. Consequently, many of these toxins are not eliminated, and end up stored in body tissues and organs. Repeated exposure to these poisons increases levels of toxicity in the body and interferes with normal organ functioning, which further impedes the body's processes of detoxification. In addition, toxic substances can interact within the body to form even more dangerous chemicals.

Basically, toxins cause disease by irritating cells. They provoke changes in individual cells and in DNA structure, which is the genetic code for cellular reproduction. This means that the blueprint for healthy cell reproduction has been tampered with, and as a result, all new cells that are created are abnormal. In addition, exposure to toxins weakens the immune system. Our bodies have the ability to eliminate damaged or abnormal cells and to repair damaged DNA, but if the immune system is weakened or there is an overload of chemical assaults on the body, the stage is set for degenerative disease to take root. Through practices of detoxification, you are giving your body the opportunity to come back into balance so that your immune system functions optimally, unhealthy cells are eliminated, and your cellular blueprints are restored to a healthy state.

Creating a Healthy Environment

The toxicity of our bodies is a direct reflection of the toxicity of our external environment. As the Earth has become more polluted, so have our bodies. In essence, we have become giant filters for all of the environmental toxins that we come into contact with. Our physical, mental, emotional, and spiritual health suffers greatly as a result. Optimally, we will restore our well-being by restoring the health of our home, the Earth. For true healing to occur, we must acknowledge our sacred connection to the Earth and learn to live in harmony with our environment.

For many people, the first step of awakening to this connection is a desire to improve personal health. When we take conscious action to improve our personal well-being, we naturally begin to be more aware of how we live our daily lives. By making the effort to live in a conscious manner, you are creating a life that is healthy not only for yourself, but for the Earth and all of its inhabitants. Making mindful changes in the way that you live is empowering and life-affirming.

The following five steps are the primary ways that you can create a healthy lifestyle to support your detoxification efforts. Remember, the fewer toxins you are exposed to, the fewer toxins that your body has to cope with.

THE FIVE ESSENTIAL PRINCIPLES OF A HEALTHFUL LIFESTYLE

Principle #1: Eat Organic Foods

Pesticides, herbicides, and other poisonous chemicals used by the agricultural industry are a primary cause of toxicity to our bodies and to the Earth. You've heard it before, but it bears repeating:

You are what you eat. Our cells—the building blocks of our bodies—are created from the foods that we take in. Decide now to become conscious of every bite of food that you put into your body. If you are like most people, you probably eat something, a meal or a snack, several times each day. Every time you eat, you are either building healthy cells and vibrant well-being, or you are adding to the load of toxins that your body has to process.

Virtually every one of us carries residues of pesticides and other chemicals stored in our fat tissues. These poisons enter our food supply in a variety of ways. Synthetic fertilizers, pesticides, and other agricultural chemicals are applied to crops, and animals raised for the dairy and meat industries are fed hormones, antibiotics, and other chemical cocktails. During food processing, a huge array of chemicals are added to foods to flavor, sweeten, color, preserve, bleach, and texturize the ingredients beyond recognition. Even food packaging contains toxins that leach into the contents, such as the lead or aluminum in cans, and the polyvinyl chloride in the plastic wrap used to package meats, poultry, and fish. All of these unnatural substances end up in our bodies.

Creating a Health-Supportive Diet

There are a few simple steps that will greatly reduce your exposure to toxins in food. Make it a point to eat fresh foods in season. Fresh fruits and vegetables provide an abundance of vitamins and minerals and protective antioxidants. Less processed foods also contain fewer additives. Most important is to buy only organically grown produce. Fruits and vegetables are treated with a large variety of toxic pesticides, fumigants, fungicides, and fertilizers. Washing or even peeling produce does not remove the vast majority of these chemicals. Many chemicals applied to fruits and vegetables become part of the cells of the plant, and then become part of your cells when you eat them.

If you eat meat, buy that which is labeled as organically raised or free range, or at least buy poultry and meats that have not been given hormones or other drugs. Meats, poultry, and fish are high on the food chain and concentrate large amounts of toxins in their flesh. Eating fish provides significant health benefits, but avoid swordfish, which concentrates large amounts of mercury, and fish and shellfish from coastal waters where contamination is likely. In addition, think of animal protein as an accompaniment to your meal instead of as the centerpiece. Three to four ounces of meat, poultry, or fish once or twice daily provides an abundant amount of protein. You might also consider experimenting with one or two meatless days a week, substituting vegetable proteins such as tofu, tempeh, or beans. Vegetarians incur significantly less cancer, heart disease, and other degenerative diseases than meat eaters for a number of reasons. A vegetarian diet tends to be high in fiber, low in fat, and rich in antioxidants and other protective nutrients that vegetables and fruits provide. I do not advocate a strict vegetarian diet because everyone is unique, and people vary in their dietary needs. While some do fine as vegetarians, others fare much better when they include animal protein in their diet. If you do eat animal protein, still concentrate on making vegetables and fruits the most important part of your diet. They provide an abundance of nutrients that purify and protect every cell of your body.

Make an effort to eat a varied diet by expanding your food choices. Most people get into dietary ruts, eating the same foods day after day. By making a conscious effort to eat a wide variety of foods, you lessen your exposure to the toxins that might be in any one particular food. In addition, broadening your food choices provides you with a greater abundance of vitamins, minerals, antioxidants, and as yet undiscovered nutrients that support your optimal health.

PRINCIPLES OF A HEALTH-SUPPORTIVE DIET

Eat organically grown foods

Emphasize fresh fruits and vegetables

Minimize processed foods

Reduce animal proteins

Avoid unnecessary packaging

Eat a varied diet

A wonderful benefit of undergoing a purification program is that you will become more attuned to your body's needs. If you listen, your body will tell you exactly what you need to eat for optimal health. Cultivate the habit of checking in with yourself to find out what will best nourish you. Be flexible and open, accepting that your needs will fluctuate from day to day, depending on your activities, the season, and normal variations in hormones and other metabolic processes. For more specific guidelines for creating an optimal health-supportive diet, see Chapter 13.

Finding Organic Foods

Twenty years ago, organically grown commercial foods were virtually unheard of. Today, there is a cornucopia of every food imaginable being organically grown, and an entire industry has evolved to meet the demand for organic foods. In my travels around the country, I have found that organically grown foods are increasingly available. Natural foods stores generally have the best selection of organic grains, beans, pasta, breads, dairy products, oils, and other staples, but even many large supermarket chains carry a decent selection of organic foods. Look for the label "certified organic," which indicates that the food has been grown and processed without the use of synthetic chemicals. "Natural" does not mean organic. When buying packaged foods, look not only for organic ingredients, but also check to see that the product does not contain artificial preservatives, flavors, colors, or other additives. Avoid any products made with hydrogenated or partially hydrogenated oils, which are toxic to the liver and detrimental to your health. Avoid unnecessary packaging, and if you buy canned foods, make certain that the can is marked "lead free."

Well-stocked natural foods stores also offer a selection of fresh organic fruits and vegetables. Organic produce is often more expensive than regular produce, but it's worth the extra money. Washing conventionally grown produce removes only the surface residues of chemicals at best. Many of the poisons used by the agricultural industry are systemic—they become part of the fruit or vegetable, and then part of your body. Studies have proven that organically grown fruits and vegetables contain more vitamins and minerals than conventionally grown produce. And organic produce tastes better.

Ideally, grow some or all of your own vegetables and fruits. Not only do you have control over every aspect of how the plant is grown, but your energy intermingles with the energy of the plant, and you are connected with your source of nourishment from the time you plant the seeds until you harvest the plant. Don't let lack of space for a large garden deter you. A small garden space—or even a couple of large pots—can provide you with tender organic salad greens in the spring and hearty kale, collard, and mustard greens in the fall. Farmer's markets are also often wonderful sources of locally grown organic produce, and even some conventional supermarkets are beginning to carry organic produce. Become an advocate for organic foods—ask your local supermarket produce manager to stock organic fruits and vegetables. Don't be afraid to ask for what you want! The organic foods movement is blossoming because consumers are demanding healthful, good quality, nontoxic foods.

If your local shopping situation is bleak and doesn't show promise of change, consider shopping by mail-order. There are excellent companies that specialize in shipping a beautiful variety of organic foods—including fresh produce—right to your front door. See the Resource section for companies that provide organic produce and other foods by mail-order. The time that you spend locating organic foods is well worth the effort. Organically grown foods are an investment in your health, and in the health of the Earth, too.

Principle # 2: Drink Pure Water

Water is the river of life, flowing through every cell of our bodies, cleansing and renewing us constantly. Although we seem to be made up of dense muscle and bone, our bodies are approximately 60 percent water. Water is essential for our survival. If necessary, we can go for weeks or even months without food, but for only three or four days without water.

Tragically, we have polluted virtually every source of water available to us. Toxins flow into our drinking water from industrial and agricultural runoff, animal wastes, heavy metal mining, land fills and chemical dumps, acid rain, leaking septic tanks and inadequate sewage treatment facilities, and metals and plastic molecules that leach from pipes that transport water. Our drinking water has been found to contain a staggering variety of more than two thousand toxic chemicals. These chemicals are not removed by most water treatment facilities. The primary purpose of a water treatment facility is to disinfect the water, and most facilities use chlorine to eradicate any disease causing microorganisms such as bacteria, viruses, and protozoans. But chlorine is also toxic, and is suspected of damaging the immune system and contributing to heart disease. In addition, chlorine combines with other contaminants in water to form powerful cancer-causing substances.

Not only do we take in water pollutants through drinking and cooking, but we also take in significant amounts through bathing. Your skin is permeable and readily absorbs into your bloodstream approximately 60 percent of whatever is applied to it. The amount of toxins your skin takes in during a 15-minute bath or shower is approximately equal to drinking 1 quart or more of the same water! Even breathing the fumes of volatile chemicals such as chlorine from running water is hazardous to your health. As well as being detrimental to your health, chlorine is extremely drying to your hair and skin.

Finding Pure Water

Until we clean up our precious water resources, the most practical answer for obtaining pure water is to filter the water that you use in your home. Many people buy bottled water, but the water you are paying for may be no better than the water that comes out of your tap. If you must buy bottled water, buy it in glass or hard clear plastic containers. Avoid buying or storing water in soft translucent plastic jugs. Molecules of soft plastic dissolve easily into water, and plastic is highly toxic.

Far superior to buying bottled water is to invest in a good home water purifier. There are a number of different water purifiers on the market. The majority use activated carbon as a filtration medium, which is an excellent chemical adsorbant. Instead of absorbing toxins, each particle of carbon has many microscopic surfaces that capture, or *adsorb*, toxic chemicals. Activated carbon removes chlorine and a significant number of other contaminants, depending on the quality of the filter. Water purifiers with solid carbon block filters are better at removing contaminants than granulated carbon filters. Replace the carbon filter at least as often as recommended by the manufacturer, because when the filter is saturated with toxins, it no longer purifies your water. More elaborate home water purification systems include reverse osmosis, where the water is forced through a semi-permeable membrane that filters contaminants, and steam distillation, which removes contaminants by heating water to boiling and capturing the condensed steam. Carbon water filters are also available for attaching to the shower to provide a chemical-free bath. And when traveling, I always carry a small portable carbon filter to ensure that I have clean drinking and cooking water wherever I go.

Principle #3: Breathe Clean Air

Air pollution is an inescapable hazard of modern life; air pollutants are carried on wind currents around the world to places far from the source of origin. Estimates by the Environmental Protection Agency show that more than half of the U. S. population is breathing toxic levels of air pollutants. These pollutants harm the respiratory system, poison the blood, and damage the genetic structure of cells. Asthma, bronchitis, emphysema, allergies, cardiovascular disease, lung cancer, and headaches are all linked to toxins in the air. While air pollution is everywhere, it makes sense to make every effort to live in as nonpolluted an area as possible. Even within the same town or city, there are locations that are less polluted than others. Areas with abundant trees and shrubs and locations near water tend to have cleaner air. Wherever you live, you can provide your cells with a much-needed boost of oxygen by spending as much time as possible in parks, gardens, wooded areas, or by the waterfront.

Another disturbing fact of modern life is that the level of indoor pollutants in many homes is often higher than the polluted air outdoors. The current practice of tightly sealing homes to make them energy efficient creates the perfect environment for the accumulation of toxins. The synthetic materials used in building and furnishing most homes also contain numerous toxins and are a primary source of indoor pollutants. Other common household pollutants include fumes from gas appliances, tobacco smoke, aerosol sprays, paints, solvents, moth crystals, household cleaning products, pesticides, formaldehyde-treated building materials and fabrics, soft plastics such as shower curtains, and gardening chemicals.

For optimal health, strive to make your home environment as healthy as possible. While you might not have a lot of control over the outdoor pollutants you are exposed to, you do have a great deal of control over the pollutants in your home. Begin by replacing synthetic products or chemicals with nontoxic alternatives. For every item you buy, think natural! Following are general suggestions for reducing indoor toxins and creating a healthy home environment. For more ideas, see the Resource section.

Purifying Your Home Environment

To reduce the level of pollutants that may accumulate within your home, open the windows daily to allow fresh air to circulate. If you live with a smoker or live in a heavily polluted area, installing an air purifier is a good idea. Air filters can be installed in the ventilation system of the house or portable air filters can be used in individual rooms. One of the most aesthetically pleasing methods of air filtration is to fill your home with living plants. Tests by NASA have shown that through their natural process of photosynthesis, common houseplants remove a variety of pollutants from the air, especially gases such as carbon monoxide, formaldehyde, carbon dioxide, and benzene. Philodendrons, spider plants, scheffleras, chrysanthemums, ferns, and dracaena are all excellent air filters. The more the better, but plan on using several medium-sized plants per room for optimal air purification.

Substitute natural materials for synthetics whenever possible. Buy solid wood furniture instead of particle board or plastic. Upholster furniture with natural fabrics instead of synthetics, and use natural fillings such as down or wool instead of foam. Use only nontoxic cleaning products throughout your home, and make an effort to find the healthiest alternative to common toxins such as paints, solvents, and pesticides. There are many nontoxic solutions available today. Check the Resource section for suggestions.

Creating a Healthful Kitchen

Making healthful meals begins with creating a healthy kitchen environment. Make sure your kitchen has good air circulation, and have any gas appliances checked for leaks. Replace nonstick or aluminum pots, pans, and baking dishes with cast iron, glass, stainless steel, or enamel cookware. Use wooden cutting boards (which have been proven to have natural antibacterial properties) and wooden or stainless steel cooking utensils instead of plastic. Avoid plastics whenever possible, including plastic storage containers, plastic bags, and plastic wrap. All soft plastics leach harmful molecules into foods, and when heated, release plastic molecules into the air. Use glass food storage containers, cloth or mesh bags, and parchment or waxed paper instead. Install a good water filter for a clean source of drinking and cooking water. Substitute nontoxic vegetable-based dish soaps and cleansers for chemical products. See the Resource section for ideas for making your own natural cleaning products, including natural substitutes for highly toxic products such as oven cleaners.

Making Your Bathroom Into a Spa

Begin by replacing your plastic shower curtain with a tightly woven cloth curtain. The unpleasant plastic odor that emanates from vinyl shower curtains is vinyl chloride, a poisonous chemical that has been linked to cancer and chronic respiratory problems. Install an activated carbon water filter on your shower to remove chlorine, which is absorbed into your skin and creates hazardous fumes. Replace synthetic towels and bath rugs with those made of cotton. The purest towels and rugs are those made from natural, untreated, unbleached cotton. Instead of synthetic air fresheners, open the windows, or use natural essential oil sprays or aromatherapy candles. Substitute natural vegetable-based tub, tile, and toilet cleansers for toxic chemical products.

Creating a Pure Sleeping Environment

You spend almost one-third of your life in bed, and much of your body's regeneration and deep-cleansing work takes place while you sleep. It makes sense to make your bedroom a safe haven from toxins. Most conventional mattresses are made with polyurethane foam, which releases poisonous chemicals into the air for years. The healthiest bed to sleep on is one made from natural cotton, such as a simple futon or a mattress made with spring coils and stuffed with cotton batting. At the very least, treat yourself to 100 percent untreated, unbleached cotton sheets. Avoid "no-iron" or "easy care" sheets. They are impregnated with a permanent formaldehyde finish that envelops you in toxins each night. Formaldehyde is a carcinogen, and causes symptoms of toxicity such as fatigue, insomnia, headaches, nausea, respiratory irritation, and skin rashes.

Once you experience the silky comfort of natural cotton sheets, you'll never want to sleep on synthetic blend sheets again. Natural cotton flannel sheets are a cozy and healthful option for winter. To outfit the rest of your bed, choose natural blankets made from cotton or wool, or down-filled comforters. Replace synthetic foam pillows with pillows stuffed with down, wool, or cotton. Keep fresh air circulating in your bedroom, particularly at night. Even during the coldest months, keep a window open an inch or two. You'll sleep better, and awaken refreshed.

CREATING A HEALTHFUL HOME

Avoid plastics

Avoid aluminum and nonstick cookware

Avoid household and garden chemicals

Avoid synthetic carpets and upholstery

Avoid particle board furniture

Install water filters in kitchen and bath

Use stainless steel, glass, or ceramic cookware

Use nontoxic cleaning supplies

Open your windows

Fill your home with plants

Buy cotton bedding and towels

Use natural fabrics on furniture

Buy solid wood furniture

Principle #4: Avoid Other Common Toxins

While eating organic foods, drinking pure water, and breathing clean air provide a good foundation for health, it is also important to cultivate awareness of other toxins that permeate modern life. While some of these harmful substances come as no surprise— tobacco, for example—others, such as synthetic shampoos and body lotions, may not be products that you generally think of as hazardous to your health. But they are, because any chemical that you inhale, ingest, apply to your body, or otherwise come into contact with must be neutralized and metabolized by the liver and the other organs of detoxification. With this in mind, it makes sense to be aware of all harmful chemicals in your environment, to make an effort to eliminate your exposure to them and to find more healthful alternatives.

Tobacco—A Known Health Hazard

Tobacco in all forms is obviously highly toxic. Tobacco smoke and many of the poisons found in it are known carcinogens. If you smoke, make every effort to quit. If you live with a smoker, try to institute a policy of outdoor smoking only, or confine smoking to one room of the house and keep the door to that room closed. In addition, install good air filters throughout your home to create as smoke-free an environment as possible.

Avoid frequenting public places where smoking is allowed, such as bars, restaurants, clubs, and coffee shops. Second hand smoke is unquestionably harmful to your health. Poisons such as lead, arsenic, formaldehyde, methyl chloride, and ammonia are among the toxic chemicals that are released into the environment by burning tobacco.

Cut Back on Caffeine

Caffeine is a common toxin that has become a part of daily life for many people. A cup or two—or even more—of coffee is almost a national institution for getting the day started. Because coffee is such a commonly accepted substance, the fact that caffeine is a powerful stimulant drug is often overlooked. Caffeine speeds up metabolism, raising blood pressure and heart rate. It increases symptoms of anxiety, causes insomnia, and results in fatigue after the initial stimulant effect wears off. Because caffeine overstimulates the adrenal glands, it places the body in a state of chronic stress.

Caffeine also has laxative and diuretic properties, which causes nutrients such as calcium to be leached from the body. Osteoporosis, PMS and menopausal problems, and fibrocystic breast disease are all made worse by caffeine. I have worked with many women who experienced dramatic improvement in PMS symptoms and breast tenderness simply by relinquishing their morning cup of coffee.

Caffeine is highly addictive, as anyone who has tried to kick a coffee habit knows. Giving up coffee causes headaches, fatigue, and irritability for several days while the body detoxifies. Stick with it, and you'll feel like a new person within a few days. Not only is caffeine found in coffee, but it also is found in black and green teas, chocolate, colas and other soft drinks, and many over-the-counter drugs such as stimulants, cold remedies, and pain medications.

If you do drink coffee, try not to drink it every day. Make sure to drink only organically grown, because coffee is subjected to a variety of poisonous chemicals during farming and processing. Decaffeinated coffee presents its own hazards. Unless it has been steam-distilled (labeled as water-processed or Swiss processed), it has been treated with highly toxic chemicals. Try substituting grain coffee or ginger tea for your usual cup of coffee. If you want a mild caffeine boost, choose organic black or green tea, which contain potent antioxidants and provide significant health benefits, unlike coffee.

Reduce Alcohol Consumption

Alcohol, in the form of beer, wine, and hard liquor, is another commonly accepted drug that many people use daily, but for relaxation instead of stimulation. As a central nervous system depressant, alcohol relieves tension and inhibitions. The moderate use of alcohol has been found to have certain health benefits, including improvement in circulation, an increase in beneficial HDL cholesterol levels, reduction of stress, and enhancement of digestion. But many people drink far more than moderate amounts of alcohol.

Alcohol is metabolized by the liver, and excessive intake can interfere with the liver's ability to detoxify other chemicals, including estrogen and other hormones. Excessive use of alcohol is a factor in cardiovascular disease, cancer, and emotional disturbances such as depression and anxiety. Alcohol also acts as a diuretic, and causes dehydration and the loss of nutrients, especially B-complex vitamins and minerals such as calcium and magnesium. In general, if you have a healthy liver and gastrointestinal system, urinary tract, and nervous system, drinking a moderate amount of alcohol should do you no harm. A moderate amount is defined as 4 ounces of wine, 12 ounces of beer, or 1 ounce of hard liquor. For optimal liver health, keep your alcohol consumption to no more than twice a week. If you drink alcohol, red wine is the best choice, since it contains health-protective benefits from the phytonutrients found in grapes. Buy organic varieties, because grapes are often heavily treated with chemicals.

Substitute Natural Remedies for Synthetic Drugs

All drugs—including prescription, over-the-counter, and recreational—are also toxins. They all must be metabolized by the liver and excreted by the organs of detoxification. Obviously, there are times when the use of prescription drugs is necessary. The healthier you are, however, the less need you will have for prescription drugs. The same is true for over-the-counter drugstore medications. If you find yourself running to the drugstore for pain killers, cold medications, laxatives, or sleep aids, I encourage you to explore the healthful options that are available at your natural foods store. There are many natural remedies that are as effective as drugstore medications without the unpleasant or harmful side effects.

I have relied on herbal and other natural remedies for more than twenty years to treat every imaginable type of health complaint. Not only are these remedies effective, but I like being in control of my health care and I feel a tremendous sense of satisfaction when I create my own medicines. The simple act of brewing a cup of herbal tea initiates the healing process, because all healing begins with positive intention. Herbal medicines are much more satisfying than popping a synthetic drug from the pharmacy into your mouth. Herbal medicines also work in harmony with your body. Instead of masking or suppressing symptoms, they support your body's innate healing wisdom. Remember, your body knows how to heal itself. Most of the time, the best thing you can do is to get out of the way, and to simply give your body the help it needs to do its healing work. For more information about natural home remedies, see the Resource section.

Other alternative therapies, such as acupuncture, homeopathy, massage, and chiropractic also stimulate the healing process. My primary health care practitioner is a naturopathic physician. Her emphasis is on helping my body to heal naturally, and she recommends herbs, dietary supplements, and acupuncture instead of pharmaceutical drugs. There are natural alternatives available for virtually every health problem. I strongly encourage you to work with a holistically oriented practitioner in your quest for optimal health. To find out how to locate alternative health care practitioners, see the Resource section.

Use Natural Cosmetics and Bodycare Products

Cosmetics and bodycare products are often overlooked as sources of toxins, but in reality they are a significant source of chemical exposure. Such products are used on a daily basis, and must be metabolized and neutralized by the liver. Shampoos, conditioners, body lotions, deodorants, aftershave lotions and perfumes are all used directly on the body. Although these products are applied externally and not ingested, the skin, including the scalp, absorbs approximately 60 percent of whatever substance is applied to it.

Study the labels of your bodycare products just as carefully as you read food ingredient labels. Tens of thousands of chemicals, including poisons such as aluminum, formaldehyde, and artificial colorings are used in commercial cosmetics and bodycare products. Why put anything onto your body that you wouldn't consider eating? There are many wonderful natural cosmetics and bodycare items available at natural foods stores. You can also make many of your own bodycare products simply and inexpensively from natural ingredients that you have in your kitchen with the addition of herbs and fragrant essential oils. I have been making most of my own bodycare products for years, and prefer my creations to anything I can buy. For information on making your own natural bodycare products, see the Resource section.

Principle #5: Reduce Stress

Stress is a major contributor to the creation of toxins in our bodies. It's estimated that almost 90 percent of illnesses are stress related! Under stress, the body goes into survival mode, and the adrenal glands release increased amounts of adrenaline and other hormones. These hormones raise heart rate and blood pressure and prepare the body to fight or flee. At the same time, digestion shuts down, immune activity is decreased, and muscles become tense. Every organ system is negatively affected by stress, and when the body is subjected to long-term or repeated stressors, breakdowns inevitably begin to occur. In addition, stress creates free radicals, which are mutant molecules that cripple healthy cells. Free radicals have been identified as a primary cause of degenerative disease and aging. Learning to manage stress is one of the most important steps you can take to protect your health.

While a certain amount of stress is normal and stimulates alertness and productivity, too much stress is definitely harmful to your well-being. Stress can be defined as your personal internal reactions to external life events. Your particular emotional makeup and your current coping mechanisms determine to a large extent the way that you handle stressful events. Some people are unfazed by virtually any difficulty that comes their way, while others live in a constant state of anxiety. If you frequently feel overwhelmed, irritable, anxious, or depressed, you can benefit greatly from stress-management techniques. Take the time to learn and practice simple breathing, meditation, and relaxation exercises to help restore your body to a healthy balance. For specific breathing and relaxation techniques that relieve stress and promote well-being, see Chapter 16. In addition, cultivate supportive, loving relationships, and spend time doing things that bring you pleasure. On a physical level, regular exercise, sufficient sleep and rest, and good nutrition help to buffer the effects of stress.

Creating Joy

Lowering the level of stress in your life is a positive step toward the creation of health. Begin by identifying life situations that cause you emotional stress. What makes you feel tense or unhappy? Make a promise to yourself to change anything in your life that doesn't bring you joy. Stress and joy cannot exist at the same time. The more joy you have in your life, the healthier you will be. If you are carrying around the idea that life has to be difficult, this is a perfect opportunity to rethink that belief. This does not mean that you will not encounter difficult situations in life. But embrace your power to change the things that are within your capacity to change, and ask for support in the changes that you want to make. As for the things that you cannot change, remember that you can transform your approach and your attitude, which is immensely stress-relieving.

A life-changing stress-management technique is to learn to identify attitudes which contribute to stress, and to practice healthier ways of thinking. Therapy can be a powerful tool for helping you to break free from thinking patterns that are stressful and emotionally toxic. A good therapist can help you to identify these toxic emotions, and can provide skillful support along the path of emotional cleansing and healing. See Chapter 17 for specific ways of transforming life attitudes which cause distress.

HOW TO REDUCE STRESS

Practice deep-breathing exercises

Practice relaxation exercises

Cultivate loving relationships

Exercise regularly

Get sufficient sleep and rest

Eat a healthy diet

Identify and change stressful attitudes

Do what brings you joy

chapter five

Seven Powerful Ways to Help Your Body Cleanse

Creating a nontoxic environment and lifestyle are essential for optimal health. At the same time, no matter how pristine your environment, your body still needs to detoxify on daily basis. There are a number of powerful and effective ways of assisting your body in the process of purification. These practices will support your overall health and well-being, while helping you to feel younger and more vibrantly alive. The principles presented here are addressed in detail in Chapters 12 through 17.

Cleansing Principle #1: Detoxify with Herbs

Herbs have been used for centuries for cleansing and detoxification. All traditional systems of healing include specific herbs to aid in purification of the body. These herbs are generally used as part of a cleansing program one or more times a year to keep the body in optimal health. Cleansing herbs are also prescribed during times of sickness to help the body to recover from disease. By supporting the organs of elimination, herbs facilitate the process of purification.

Purifying herbs stimulate the elimination of wastes, increase urination, encourage perspiration, stimulate circulation, enhance immune functioning, cleanse excess mucus from the lungs and intestines, and improve digestion. A balanced herbal cleansing program supports each organ system of detoxification—the large intestine, the liver, the kidneys, the lymphatic system, the skin, and the lungs. Herbal cleansing formulas are also designed to ameliorate any possible side effects of cleansing. During a cleansing program, it's helpful to use a variety of herbs both internally and externally to aid your body in the process of detoxification. With the information and recipes in Chapter 12, you can create your own herbal purification formulas tailored specifically to your needs.

Cleansing Principle #2: Eat a Cleansing Diet

The dietary choices you make play a critical role in your program of detoxification. A purifying diet is based primarily on fresh, organic vegetables and fruits. Vegetables and fruits have the greatest cleansing power of any foods. They are rich in fiber, which helps to sweep out intestinal debris. They also are the most abundant food sources of vitamins and minerals, particularly the protective antioxidants which help to neutralize free-radical damage. Free radicals are unstable molecules that damage healthy cells and cause disease and premature aging. By saturating your tissues and cells with antioxidants from fresh vegetables and fruits, you can help your body prevent and repair free-radical damage.

Cleansing diets are most effective when they are designed for your particular body type and current health condition. Other factors, such as the climate you live in, should also be taken into consideration. For example, while a juice fast may be a healthy choice for a person living in Florida who is overweight and eats a diet rich in meats and fats, the same fast would be disastrous for a vegetarian living in New England in the winter. Fasting is the most intense cleansing diet and is not appropriate for everyone. Cleansing diets should be purifying without being debilitating. In general, a gentle, gradual approach to detoxification results in deeper cleansing than a more radical program.

Along with an abundance of vegetables and fruits, detoxification diets can include nourishing soups, whole grains, healthy oils such as olive oil and flax oil, and moderate amounts of lean proteins, including animal protein for people who need extra nourishment.

Foods to avoid while on a purification program include fatty foods, excessive protein, excessive salt, sweets, refined and processed foods, flour products, and dairy products. These foods tend to create stagnation in the body, and are best abstained from during a cleanse.

While cleansing, focus on making foods light, nourishing, and easy to digest. Also practice conscious awareness at meals so that you are eating when you are hungry and stopping before you are full. This promotes the healthy development of digestive fire, or *agni*, as it is referred to in Ayurvedic medicine. Agni not only stimulates digestion, but also burns up toxic accumulations in the digestive tract. Liquid intake is important during a detoxification program. Drinking plenty of pure water and cleansing herbal teas stimulates kidney function and helps to flush wastes out of the body.

Certain dietary supplements are also useful as part of a cleansing program. I especially recommend taking antioxidants such as vitamin C, which helps to stimulate detoxification, and herbs that support healthy liver function, such as milk thistle. See Chapter 13 for specific information on purifying foods and dietary supplements, along with recommendations for designing a cleansing diet.

Cleansing Principle #3: Exercise to Enhance Detoxification

Exercise is an essential component of a detoxification program. Regular exercise increases circulation, which stimulates blood flow throughout the body and brings nutrients and oxygen to cells while carrying away toxins. The contraction of muscles is also the primary mechanism by which lymphatic fluid is moved through the lymphatic channels. Walking, bicycling, swimming, and dancing are excellent whole body exercises that stimulate circulation and lymphatic flow.

Cultivate the habit of moving as much as possible in your life. Look for every opportunity to enjoy the beautiful body that you have been blessed with. Your body craves movement, and becomes sluggish without daily exercise. Exercise promotes healthy digestion and intestinal function, enhances immune activity, keeps muscles toned and bones strong, improves mental functioning, and relieves stress and anxiety. Regular daily exercise is your best insurance for a long and healthy life. Give yourself the gift of at least 30 minutes of exercise daily, and take frequent exercise breaks throughout the day. In only 5 or 10 minutes, you can refresh your body and mind with a quick walk or a few stretching exercises. Gentle aerobic exercise such as walking oxygenates the body and alleviates stagnation. Stretching exercises and yoga open up the subtle channels of energy flow and stimulate healthy organ function.

For more information on incorporating exercise into your cleansing program and instructions for a variety of simple purifying yoga and stretching exercises, see Chapter 14.

Cleansing Principle #4: Purify with Breathing Exercises

Breathing is an involuntary act that primarily occurs beneath the level of your conscious awareness. By focusing your attention on your breath, you can dramatically affect your well-being. Special breathing exercises have been practiced in the Far East for centuries as a means of purification and renewal, and are used to heal the body, improve mental concentration, and enhance spiritual practices. The regular practice of calming breathing exercises has been proven in research studies to be an excellent method for relieving stress and anxiety.

Each time you inhale, you bring life-giving oxygen into your body, which carries nutrients to your cells and helps to purify them. With each exhalation, you eliminate toxic carbon dioxide from your bloodstream. Most people breathe shallowly and rapidly, filling only the upper portion of the lungs with oxygen. This causes a chronic, low-level state of stagnation which creates fatigue, poor concentration, headaches, and a general feeling of grogginess. Proper breathing enlivens the body and is essential for optimal health. Through the regular practice of simple breathing exercises, you can relieve tension and anxiety and help your body to cleanse with each breath you take. Chapter 16 provides instructions for a variety of cleansing and healing breathing exercises.

Cleansing Principle #5: Detoxify with Hydrotherapy

Hydrotherapy is one of the most enjoyable aspects of a detoxification program. This ancient method of purification includes saunas, steams, and herbal and aromatherapy baths. Hydrotherapy treatments increase circulation, promote relaxation, and encourage detoxification through perspiration.

The use of alternating hot and cold showers or baths stimulates circulation and promotes healthy oxygen flow to all of the cells of the body. Dry body brushing and body scrubs enhance lymphatic drainage and remove dead skin cells from the surface of the body. Steam baths and saunas increase core body temperature and promote perspiration, helping to discharge toxins from deep within the tissues and bringing them to the surface for elimination. Sauna therapy is used frequently in medical detoxification programs to help people who suffer from the effects of heavy metal, pesticide, and other toxic chemical exposure. Mineral and aromatherapy baths are soothing and aromatic treatments for promoting gentle detoxification and relaxation, and can be used regularly to help your body cleanse. See Chapter 15 for a variety of luxurious hydrotherapy treatments you can create at home.

Cleansing Principle #6: Massage Away Toxins

Massage is another delightful component of a detoxification program. A full-body massage stimulates lymphatic flow and drainage, enhances circulation, breaks up fatty deposits and cellulite, and promotes relaxation and a feeling of overall well-being. Plan to treat yourself to a weekly massage while undergoing a purification program. A professional massage is a wonderful experience, and so is exchanging massage with a friend or your partner. You can also easily perform simple self-massage routines. Massaging your body while in the bath or during a sauna or steam treatment enhances the detoxifying benefits of both. For directions for simple self-massage treatments, see Chapter 16.

Cleansing Principle #7: Detoxify Your Thinking

Your habitual patterns of thinking play a powerful role in your physical, mental, emotional, and spiritual well-being. Detoxifying your thinking is one of the most potent tools you have for healing on every level. With the help of simple exercises such as journal writing and a commitment to change, you can become aware of negative thoughts and learn to think in a self-affirming way.

Other methods of mental purification include meditation and visualization. Regular meditation has been proven to have significant health benefits, as the simple process of sitting and quieting the mind helps to bring the body into balance. Even 15 minutes of meditation daily can greatly lower stress levels, which in turn reduces the formation of toxic stress hormones. With visualization, you harness the power of your mind to create a desired outcome. All action begins with an image in the mind, and when you consciously create mental images of well-being, you support your body's natural desire for health. For an exploration of exercises in meditation and visualization and detoxifying your thinking, see Chapter 17.

PART TWO

YOUR BODY'S PATHWAYS OF DETOXIFICATION

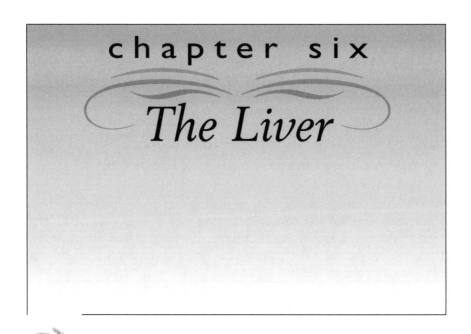

chapter six

The Liver

Your Body's Master Alchemist

Of all of the body's organs of cleansing, the liver reigns as king in the complex process of detoxification. Residing just beneath your ribs in the upper right side of your abdomen, your liver weighs about three pounds and is the largest internal organ. Working steadily day and night, the liver performs a myriad of duties—more than 500 different tasks come under the auspices of this hardworking organ!

A constant supply of blood flowing through the hepatic artery and the portal vein brings both nutrients and toxins to the liver. The liver metabolizes, stores, and distributes nutrients throughout the body. It transforms fats and proteins into glucose, the energy source for all of the cells of the body. When energy is needed, the liver releases glucose into the bloodstream. If the liver is stressed, it can have difficulties maintaining proper blood-sugar balance, which can manifest as fatigue or hypoglycemia. The liver also stores vitamins and minerals and metabolizes vitamins A, D, E, K and B-12. It manufactures bile, a fluid that aids in the digestion of fats, and stores it in the gall bladder. In addition, the liver plays an important part in the production and breakdown of blood and also makes antibodies for the immune system. In its critical role of cleansing, the liver detoxifies metabolic by-products and filters the blood to remove impurities. The liver is like a wizard in a laboratory, magically transforming toxic substances into harmless materials which can then be excreted by the organs of elimination.

While the liver is perfectly designed to protect our bodies from harmful substances, it was never meant to take on the herculean task of filtering the staggering array of new toxins that have appeared in the past century. Pesticides, solvents, toxic chemicals, drugs, and food additives are all new stressors that threaten the well-being of your liver. Valiantly, the liver struggles to keep up with its work load, but under such adverse conditions, often falls behind in its tasks. The result? Fatigue, headaches, irritability, digestive disturbances, fuzzy thinking, menstrual difficulties, and allergies—these are just a few of your liver's cries for help.

For example, the liver is responsible for helping to metabolize and eliminate excess estrogen. It transforms estrogen from its more potent forms, *estradiol* and *estrone*, to a weaker form, *estriol*. This is then passed into the bile which flows into the digestive tract for elimination through the large intestine. If liver function is compromised, it may not be able to efficiently detoxify estrogen. This results in high levels of estrogen circulating throughout the body in the bloodstream. Excess estrogen is a primary cause of menstrual difficulties and menopausal problems, and contributes to fibroid tumors, endometriosis, breast cancer, and uterine cancer.

SYMPTOMS OF POOR LIVER FUNCTION

Fatigue

Irritability

Depression

Poor concentration

Allergies

PMS

Menopausal difficulties

Headaches

Indigestion

Constipation

Hypoglycemia

Because the liver plays a role in so many biological functions, a wide variety of physical and emotional symptoms are linked to poor liver function.

If you experience symptoms of serious liver malfunction, such as jaundice, consult your health care practitioner.

The Key to Liver Rejuvenation

Here's the good news: Your liver has remarkable powers of rejuvenation, and is constantly renewing itself. The liver is so critically important that if even 90 percent were to be removed, the remaining 10 percent could regenerate itself entirely. By attending to the well-being of this vital organ, you can help to restore your liver to optimal functioning. Your overall state of health will benefit tremendously as a result.

Reducing your exposure to toxins is one of the most important things you can do to protect your liver. The fewer toxins you take in, the fewer toxins your liver has to deal with. Take a look around your environment, and see how many ways you can eliminate harmful substances in your daily life. Remember, every chemical or poison you encounter must be detoxified by your liver. Make a commitment to eat a healthy, nontoxic diet. The liver has difficulty metabolizing and detoxifying pesticides and other poisons in chemically treated foods. As a result, these toxins are stored in the body instead of being eliminated. The solution is clear: Eat organic foods, drink pure water, and avoid other dietary toxins such as alcohol, tobacco, caffeine, drugs, sugars and processed foods. The liver is also especially stressed by unhealthy fats: the saturated fats found in red meats, whole milk dairy products, and tropical vegetable oils such as palm kernel oil and coconut oil; polyunsaturated vegetable oils such as safflower, corn, soy, and sunflower oils; and hydrogenated fats such as margarine and shortenings.

While you should avoid unhealthy fats, good quality dietary fats are essential for healthy liver function and for maintaining optimal well-being. The healthiest dietary fats are extra-virgin olive oil, flax oil, and the natural oils found in fresh raw nuts and seeds. For more information on oils and fats, see Chapter 13. Olive oil in particular appears to have significant health benefits, including helping to increase levels of beneficial HDL cholesterol while lowering levels of harmful LDL cholesterol. Studies have shown that populations with a high intake of olive oil have a lower incidence of degenerative diseases such as cardiovascular disease and cancer. Naturopathic physicians frequently prescribe an olive oil "liver and gall bladder flush" to cleanse the liver during a detoxification program. This is accomplished by drinking a beverage made from olive oil, citrus juice, and pungent herbs such as garlic, ginger, and cayenne pepper first thing in the morning for 1 to 5 days. The rationale behind a liver and gall bladder flush is that by taking this mixture on an empty stomach, the liver is stimulated to dump stored toxins into the bile so that they can then be eliminated through the intestinal tract. No food should be eaten before drinking the liver flush beverage, and you should abstain from eating for 2 to 3 hours following the flush. Do drink herbal teas and pure water to help your body eliminate the toxins that are being cleansed from your liver.

Liver and Gall Bladder Flush

Mix the following ingredients in a blender:

Juice of 1 sweet grapefruit *or* 2 oranges

Juice of 1-2 lemons *or* limes

2 tablespoons extra-virgin olive oil

1 teaspoon freshly grated ginger root *or*

1-2 cloves raw garlic

pinch of cayenne pepper *or*

freshly ground black pepper

Potent Liver Cleansers Straight from the Garden

The liver's favorite foods are fresh green vegetables—preferably those with a slightly bitter taste. Dandelion greens, watercress, and mustard greens are examples of bitter greens that stimulate bile flow and help to cleanse the liver. Eating bitter greens in the springtime is a folk remedy rooted in the intuitive knowledge of what keeps the liver healthy. People in traditional cultures all over the world have eagerly sought out the first sprouts of wild greens in early spring. They know that a portion of bitter wild greens is the perfect remedy for the sluggishness caused by a long winter of sedentary living and a diet of rich, heavy, cooked foods. If you're feeling sluggish, try eating a portion of bitter greens daily. Bitter greens stimulate the flow of bile, which naturally cleanses the liver and improves digestive function.

Bob, a friend of mine who is a chef, has a special love for rich foods and fine wines. He complained of feeling tired and bloated, and frequently took antacids to relieve attacks of indigestion. To improve his digestion, I suggested that he begin taking an herbal bitters formula before each meal, and that he eat a salad of bitter greens every day. Bob was surprised to find that these simple recommendations worked so well to relieve his digestive distress. Although he still has a fondness for rich foods, he takes his herbal bitters formula twice daily and happily creates beautiful salads from watercress, tender dandelion leaves, and arugula.

Bitter greens such as dandelion, mustard, and watercress are delicious when thinly sliced and sautéed with slivered ginger root or garlic in extra virgin olive oil. Add a squeeze of lemon just before serving to perk up the flavor. In hot weather, enjoy leafy green salads with the addition of bitter greens for a delicious and refreshing change of pace. Try endive, arugula, romaine, and watercress with a dressing made of olive oil and freshly squeezed lemon or lime juice. Or make juices from any dark leafy green combined with carrots and beets and add fresh ginger along with lemon or lime for a healthy beverage that provides your liver with a concentrated dose of nutrients.

Not only is the bitter flavor found in many greens helpful for stimulating bile flow and cleansing the liver, but green leafy vegetables are rich in chlorophyll, the pigment that gives them their green color. Chlorophyll is almost identical in structure to hemoglobin, the protein in our blood that transports oxygen to the cells. Chlorophyll is thought to have a cleansing and revitalizing effect on the body, particularly the liver and the intestinal tract. Green food supplements such as *chlorella, spirulina,* and *barley grass* are rich sources of concentrated chlorophyll that can be included as part of a cleansing program. Stir 1 teaspoon of a powdered green supplement into 8 ounces of water, add a squeeze of lemon or lime, and drink first thing in the morning. In traditional Chinese medicine, the sour taste of citrus fruits is thought to nourish the liver, when taken in moderation. And according to Ayurvedic medicine, drinking warm or hot water throughout the day with a squeeze of lemon or lime juice is thought to reduce the accumulation of *ama*, or toxins, throughout the digestive tract.

CLEANSING FOODS FOR THE LIVER

Arugula

Beets

Carrots

Collard greens

Dandelion greens

Endive

Grapefruit

Kale

Lemons

Limes

Mustard greens

Parsley

Romaine

Watercress

Bitter Herbs for Liver Health

Along with bitter greens, bitter herbs are traditionally used to cleanse the liver and improve digestive function. They work by stimulating a reflex action in the digestive organs via the taste buds located at the back of the tongue. When the taste buds encounter a bitter flavor, saliva is increased and digestive secretions automatically begin to flow in the liver, gall bladder, stomach, pancreas, and small intestine. This enhances the digestion and assimilation of foods and prevents foods from stagnating in the digestive tract. By stimulating bile flow, bitter herbs help to cleanse the liver. In addition to improving digestive function, many bitter herbs have antimicrobial and antiseptic properties, which help to cleanse the digestive tract.

Herbal teas with a bitter flavor can be taken daily for a period of 3 to 6 weeks at a time as part of a purification program. Many roots have bitter properties, and are considered classic liver-cleansing herbs. Roots are traditionally prepared as *decoctions*, which means they are simmered in a covered pot over low heat for 15-20 minutes to extract the healing properties. Some of my favorite liver-cleansing herbs include burdock, dandelion, and Oregon grape root. They can be used singly or in combination as a liver-cleansing tea, and make an earthy, robust tea with a slightly bitter taste. I add fennel seeds or ginger root—or both—to improve the flavor and enhance digestion, and sometimes I add a bit of organic orange peel as well. This makes a delicious tea! I also often add licorice root as a sweetener. As part of a detoxification program, drink 3 to 4 cups daily between meals. I've found that the easiest method is to brew a large pot of tea in the morning rather than making 1 cup of tea at a time. Sip the tea warm or at room temperature throughout the day. While you can refrigerate the decoction overnight, I've found that the flavor is best when the herbs are brewed fresh each day.

Simple Liver-Cleansing Tea

2 teaspoons dandelion root

2 teaspoons Oregon grape root

1 teaspoon ginger root

1 teaspoon licorice root

3 cups water

Combine herbs and water in a covered pot. Bring to a boil, lower the heat, and simmer gently for 15 minutes. Strain, and drink 3 cups daily.

Herbal bitters tonics are a convenient way to get the benefits of bitter herbs. Combinations of bitter herbs are steeped in grain alcohol, vodka, or another alcoholic beverage for several weeks to extract the healing properties of the plants. Using 1/2 to 1 teaspoon of an herbal bitters tonic combined with warm water 15 to 30 minutes before eating stimulates the flow of digestive fluids. Bitters tonics typically include herbs such as *gentian root* that are unpleasantly bitter when prepared as a tea. There are a number of excellent bitters digestive formulas available at natural foods stores. You can also easily make your own bitters tonic with the recipe on p. 126. While most commercial digestive bitters formulas are in liquid form, some are sold as capsules. Taking bitter herbs as a liquid is much more effective than taking bitter herbs in a capsule; remember that the bitter flavor needs to come into contact with your taste buds to stimulate the flow of digestive fluids.

HERBS FOR THE LIVER

Gentian

Barberry

Yellow dock

Oregon grape

Sarsaparilla

Dandelion root

Burdock

Milk thistle

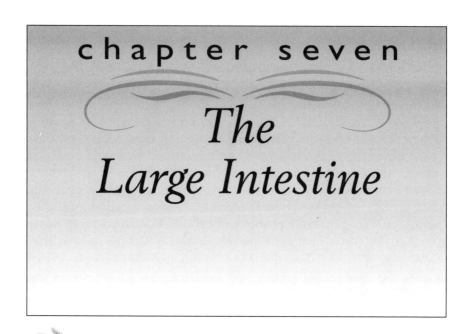

chapter seven

The Large Intestine

Your Body's Master Eliminator

The large intestine, frequently referred to as the colon, is located in the lower abdomen and is the final section of the digestive tract. Technically, the large intestine is divided into three sections: The *cecum*, which connects it to the small intestine; the *colon*, which includes the *ascending colon*, the *transverse colon*, and the *descending colon*; and the *rectum*. Waste material from the small intestine enters the large intestine at the cecum, and wends its way through the colon, five feet of hollow muscular tubing, to the rectum, where solid waste is expelled through the anus. Involuntary wavelike muscular contractions known as *peristalsis* extract fluids and move the waste through the colon. The entire process of digestion from the ingestion of food to the excretion of waste takes somewhere between 12 and 36 hours, although for some people with unhealthy colon function, wastes can remain in the body for one week or longer.

The primary function of the large intestine is to reabsorb water and minerals from waste material before it leaves the body. For most people, about 2 1/2 pints of water are reabsorbed by the colon every day. In addition, the intestinal tract is populated by an abundance of various bacteria—almost 100 different kinds—some of which synthesize essential vitamins such as B-vitamins and vitamin K, and others which protect the body against toxic microorganisms. While the large intestine is simply the pathway for the elimination of wastes, it is a key player in keeping you healthy and vital.

The most important thing you can do to keep your large intestine functioning optimally is to make sure that wastes are kept moving at a brisk pace. While some health practitioners would have you believe that intestinal function is highly individual, and that having one or two bowel movements a week is fine for some people, the truth is that for optimal health and well-being, everyone should be having one or more bowel movements a day. According to some naturopathic physicians, the ideal is to have a bowel movement after every meal, just as babies do. If you're moving your bowels at least once a day, you're probably doing just fine. But judging from the sales of laxatives in the U.S.—in excess of $400 million per year— sluggish intestines are a concern for a lot of people. Laxatives are not a healthy solution to the problem of constipation. In fact, when used regularly, they contribute to "lazy bowel syndrome," or the inability of the intestines to function without chemical stimulation.

Not only is constipation uncomfortable, but it leads to a wide range of health problems from the merely embarrassing (flatulence) to those which are life-threatening (colon cancer).

If you suffer from persistent constipation or diarrhea, a sudden change in bowel habits, or if you have blood in your stool, consult your health care practitioner.

SYMPTOMS OF COLON TOXICITY

Constipation

Flatulence

Headaches

Irritability

Abdominal distress

Diarrhea

Bad breath

Fatigue

Nausea

DISEASES RELATED TO POOR COLON FUNCTION

Diverticulosis

Diverticulitis

Hypertension

Varicose veins

Appendicitis

Irritable bowel syndrome

High blood cholesterol

Diabetes

Obesity

Autoimmune disorders

Hemorrhoids

Colon cancer

Breast cancer

Fiber: The Key to Colon Health

Getting daily exercise, drinking plenty of water, and eating a high-fiber diet is often enough to prevent and cure constipation. Karin, a friend of mine, complained of chronic long-standing constipation. She often went for a week or even longer without having a bowel movement. To help purify her system, I suggested that she follow a 2-week cleansing program. I suggested that she begin taking a teaspoon of psyllium husks daily, and eat at least 7 servings each day of fresh vegetables and fruits, especially those rich in fiber such as carrots, apples, and cabbage. I also recommended that she take *Lactobacillus acidophilus* supplements daily for 1 month to help replenish beneficial intestinal bacteria, and drink at least 6 glasses of pure water daily. Daily exercise and abdominal massage helped to stimulate intestinal function. At the end of the 2 weeks, Karin happily reported that she was having normal bowel movements each day.

A high-fiber diet provides the necessary bulk to keep waste material moving smoothly through the intestinal tract. Increasing dietary fiber increases the frequency and amount of bowel movements and decreases the toxins that are reabsorbed into the body through the large intestine. For example, fiber binds to excess estrogen and cholesterol and prevents these substances from being recirculated in the bloodstream. Fiber also encourages the growth of beneficial bacteria in the colon.

Fiber is the indigestible part of plants, and is primarily found in fruits, vegetables, whole grains, and beans. There are several different types of fiber, but they can basically be classified into two categories: *insoluble* and *soluble*. The fiber in wheat bran is an insoluble fiber, and is the most effective fiber for creating bulky, soft stools and speeding the transit of waste through the intestines. Insoluble fiber is also found in other whole grains, fruits, vegetables, nuts, and seeds. Soluble fiber is a gel-like substance that binds cholesterol and other toxins and prevents their reabsorption into the bloodstream. Oats, barley, and legumes contain soluble fiber. So do pectin-rich fruits and vegetables such as apples, bananas, citrus fruits, carrots, and cabbage. Because whole foods contain a variety of fibers, increasing your consumption of fresh vegetables and fruits, whole grains, beans, nuts, and seeds is the best approach for obtaining all of the health benefits of fiber.

HIGH-FIBER FOODS

Fresh fruits

Dried fruits

Fresh vegetables

Cooked dried beans

Nuts and seeds

Whole grains

I recommend adding supplemental fiber to your diet during a cleansing program. This supports the intestines in eliminating the larger amount of toxins that are released during detoxification, and prevents their reabsorption into the bloodstream. My favorite sources of supplemental fiber are *psyllium seed husks* and *flax seeds*. When added to water, they swell and form a gel-like substance that creates soft, bulky stools. You can buy fiber supplements that combine psyllium husks with flax seeds, pectin, guar gum, and other fibers, or you can make your own intestinal cleansing fiber blend. Take fiber supplements first thing in the morning on an empty stomach or at night just before bed. For more intensive cleansing, you can take the fiber supplement twice a day. I also often add *liquid bentonite clay* to a fiber cleansing drink. Bentonite clay is a natural mineral that has the ability to trap and bind pesticides and other toxic substances in the intestinal tract, preventing their reabsorption into the bloodstream. Be sure to drink plenty of fluids throughout the day when taking extra fiber. If you have sensitive digestion, begin with half of the recommended dose and gradually increase to the full amount if it is comfortable for you to do so.

Intestinal Cleansing Beverage

1/2 teaspoon powdered psyllium husks

1-2 tablespoons flax seeds, ground

1 tablespoon liquid bentonite clay (optional)

pinch of powdered ginger

8 ounces organic apple juice or water

Grind flax seeds in a clean coffee grinder. Add the ground flax seeds, psyllium husks, bentonite clay, and ginger to 4 ounces of apple juice or water and mix thoroughly, then add the remaining 4 ounces of liquid and stir well. Drink immediately.

Healing Foods for the Large Intestine

Not only are vegetables and fruits good sources of fiber, but many are also rich in *beta carotene*. Beta carotene keeps the mucous membranes healthy throughout the body, including the mucosal lining of the large intestine. Studies have shown that beta carotene is protective against colon cancer. Foods that are good sources of beta carotene include dark leafy greens and deep yellow-orange vegetables and fruits. In general, the deeper green or yellow-orange the fruit or vegetable is, the richer it is in beta carotene.

Cruciferous vegetables such as cabbage, broccoli, kale, collards, cauliflower, and brussels sprouts contain special compounds that stimulate enzymes which play a role in the body's natural process of detoxification. The constituents that give cruciferous vegetables their odoriferous nature encourage the production of *glutathione*, a potent antioxidant produced by the body that protects cells from free radical damage. In the intestinal tract, glutathione detoxifies rancid fats, a prime promoter of free radicals, and prevents the reabsorption of these dangerous molecules into the bloodstream.

Food and herbs with mucilagenous properties are also beneficial for the health of the large intestine. The slippery consistency of foods such as oats and barley and herbs such as aloe juice, flax seeds, fenugreek, and marshmallow root help to heal an inflamed colon and also help to restore the mucosal lining. However, if you are sensitive to gluten-containing grains, you may need to avoid oats and barley.

Beneficial bacteria such as the *Lactobacillus acidophilus* organism make their home in the walls of the intestinal tract. These friendly flora maintain a healthy internal environment by preventing the overgrowth of problem-causing microorganims such as the Candida albicans fungus. To encourage the proliferation of healthy intestinal bacteria, include sources of Lactobacillus acidophilus in your diet. Foods rich in Lactobacillus acidophilus include yogurt that contains active live cultures, miso soup, and naturally fermented and unpasteurized pickles. Lactobacillus acidophilus supplements can also be taken during a cleansing and detoxification program to help to reestablish healthy intestinal flora. Take 1 capsule with each meal, or follow the directions given by the manufacturer.

HEALING FOODS FOR THE LARGE INTESTINE

Beta-carotene rich fruits and vegetables:
Dark leafy greens
Deep yellow vegetables

Cruciferous vegetables:
Broccoli, cabbage, kale, cauliflower

Mucilagenous foods and herbs:
Oats, barley, marshmallow root, flax seeds

Friendly flora foods:
Yogurt, miso, unpasteurized pickles

Abdominal Massage for Intestinal Health

Abdominal massage helps to improve intestinal function and stimulates the movement of wastes through the large intestine. Abdominal massage can be performed daily, preferably first thing in the morning before eating. Lie down on a comfortable surface. Oil your abdomen with massage oil if desired. Place your left hand on top of your right hand, and starting at your lower right abdomen, press gently into your abdomen with your fingertips. Massage gently with a slow, circular motion, pressing as deeply as you comfortably can. Move your hands up about an inch, and repeat the circular massage movement. Continue massaging, moving up the right side of your abdomen, across the center, and down the left side, following the path of the large intestine. Finish by rubbing your abdomen with the palm of your hand in the same clockwise direction, using smooth, gliding strokes.

Stimulate Cleansing with Castor Oil Compresses

In naturopathic medicine, castor oil compresses are used to help to improve intestinal function and cleansing. You'll need a piece of cotton or wool flannel large enough so that when it is folded in half it will cover the lower abdomen. Soak the cloth in warm castor oil, wring it out so that it is saturated with the oil but not dripping, and apply to the abdomen. Cover with a cotton towel, apply a hot water bottle, and allow the compress to remain in place for 1 to 2 hours. Castor oil stains, so be sure to use an old towel, wear clothing that you don't mind staining, and protect the surface that you will be lying on.

Herbs for the Large Intestine

In addition to soothing mucilagenous herbs such as aloe juice and marshmallow, and bulk-promoting herbs such as flax seeds and psyllium husks, a number of specific herbs have laxative properties which stimulate peristalsis and can be helpful as part of a detoxification program. *Cascara sagrada* is perhaps the most gentle of the stimulant laxatives and has the reputation of helping to restore tone to the intestinal tract. I always travel with a small bottle of the tincture. It works wonders for the sluggish bowels that invariably accompany a change in routine. Take 1 dropperful of tincture in a small amount of warm water at night before sleeping. You can also make a tea from dried cascara sagrada bark. The taste is bitter, but not unpleasant. Simmer 1 teaspoon of cascara sagrada, 1/2 teaspoon of ginger root, and 1/2 teaspoon of licorice root in 1 cup of water for 15 minutes in a covered pot. Strain, and drink before bed.

HERBS FOR THE LARGE INTESTINE

Mucilagenous Herbs (To rejuvenate mucosal lining):

Marshmallow root

Slippery elm

Aloe vera juice

Oats

Flax seeds

Laxative Herbs

Psyllium seeds

Flax seeds

Dandelion root

Licorice root

Yellow dock

Cascara sagrada

Buckthorn

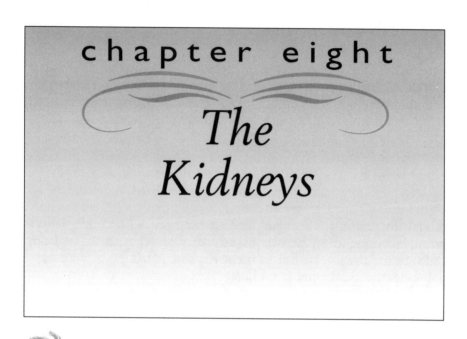

chapter eight

The Kidneys

Your Body's Master Purifier

The kidneys work in harmony with the other organs of detoxification to cleanse and purify the body. Residing in your mid-lower back, your kidneys are shaped like kidney beans, and are each approximately 4 to 6 inches long, or about the size of a fist. These small hard-working organs are responsible for filtering waste products from the entire bloodstream. Blood flows into the kidneys through the renal arteries at the rate of more than 1 quart per minute, or close to 475 gallons per day. Approximately 240 times each day, your bloodstream is purified through 1 million tiny filters within the kidneys called *nephrones*. In the unfathomable wisdom of the body, the kidneys distinguish between nutrients and waste products. Metabolic wastes such as urea from the breakdown of proteins, excess mineral salts, and toxins such as drugs are filtered from the bloodstream, while nutrients such as amino acids and glucose are returned to the body.

One of the most important functions of the kidneys is to regulate the balance of fluids in the body. Between one and two quarts of water, combined with metabolic wastes, mineral salts, and toxins, are excreted daily as urine. Through eliminating excess mineral salts in the urine, the kidneys maintain the proper balance of electrolytes in the blood—the essential minerals sodium, chloride, potassium, and magnesium. Electrolytes facilitate the conduction of minute electrical currents within the body, thus maintaining proper fluid and acid-base balance and healthy muscle and nerve function. An imbalance of electrolytes can cause fatigue, muscle weakness and loss of coordination, heart rhythm disturbances, muscle cramps, and mental confusion.

Many synthetic diuretics are dangerous because they cause the kidneys to excrete excessive amounts of electrolytes. Diuretics can be helpful to relieve water retention, such as that caused by the hormonal fluctuations that many women experience premenstrually. I often recommend an herbal diuretic to women who suffer from PMS during the week prior to menstruation. A tea made from dandelion leaf is usually my first choice.

Ava, one of my students, suffered terribly from water retention each month in the week prior to menstruation. Her breasts swelled and were very tender, her abdomen became bloated, and her fingers swelled so that she was unable to wear her wedding ring. I recommended that she begin drinking three cups of dandelion leaf tea daily at the first sign of water retention. The tea immediately eased her symptoms, and had none of the side effects of synthetic diuretics.

Dandelion leaf has been found to be as effective as pharmaceutical diuretics, but is a much safer choice because it is naturally rich in potassium and other minerals and replenishes the electrolytes that are lost through increased urination. Diuretic herbs can also be included as part of an herbal detoxification program to stimulate kidney function and to promote purification.

Signs of Kidney Distress

If the kidneys are stressed, they may have difficulty maintaining the appropriate balance of fluids in the body. This can result in water retention, with symptoms such as swollen fingers and ankles, lower back pain, and mood swings. If the kidneys are not working efficiently, they can have difficulties eliminating excess water and mineral salts, which forces the heart to work harder to pump the increased volume of blood throughout the body. Not only does this place extra stress on the heart, but it can cause a dangerous increase in blood pressure.

Indications of potential kidney or bladder disease include increased frequency of urination, a burning sensation while urinating, blood in the urine, pain in the kidney area, and water retention. If you have any of these symptoms, consult a health practitioner to determine the cause and the most appropriate course of action. Always seek prompt treatment for bladder or kidney infections to avoid possible kidney damage.

SYMPTOMS OF POOR KIDNEY FUNCTION

Water retention

Dark-colored urine

Mood swings

Kidney stones

Hypertension

Dizziness

Puffiness beneath eyes

How to Keep Your Kidneys Healthy

Poisonous residues from toxic substances such as pesticides, food additives, drugs, household and garden chemicals, solvents, and synthetic bodycare products are all filtered through the kidneys via the bloodstream. You know this by now, but it's worth repeating—to keep your organs of detoxification functioning optimally, keep your exposure to dietary and environmental toxins to a minimum.

Dietary stressors on the kidneys include alcohol, caffeine, excessive proteins and salt. Caffeine and alcohol are irritants to the urinary tract. In addition, caffeine, alcohol, and large amounts of protein all have a diuretic effect, because the kidneys are forced to work overtime to eliminate these toxins from the bloodstream. During the process, many vital minerals such as calcium and magnesium are lost as well. Coffee, alcohol, and excessive protein have all been linked to osteoporosis, kidney disease, and the formation of kidney stones.

While protein is a necessary nutrient for the growth and repair of cells, many people eat more protein than they need. For most people, 3 to 4 ounces of lean animal or vegetable protein eaten twice daily will keep the body in optimal health. When you eat more protein than you need, the excess is burned as fuel. But protein does not burn as efficiently as carbohydrates or fat, and leaves behind nitrogen wastes that have to be eliminated. The liver converts protein wastes into urea, which is sent via the bloodstream to the kidneys for excretion. Because urea is highly toxic, the kidneys work hard to eliminate it by pulling extra water from the body. This is the mechanism behind the rapid weight loss promised by proponents of high-protein low-carbohydrate diets. High-protein diets do result in quick weight loss, but the pounds lost are primarily water, not fat. Eating excessive amounts of protein places an unnecessary and harmful burden on the kidneys.

Eating too much salt can also be harmful to the kidneys. Sodium is a necessary nutrient, one that we cannot survive without. It is one of the essential electrolyte minerals, and helps to maintain healthy nerve and muscle function and to regulate the balance of fluids in the body. But excessive sodium intake can cause water retention which increases the volume of blood that the kidneys must filter. For susceptible individuals, excess salt can contribute to the development of hypertension, stroke, cardiovascular disease, and kidney disease.

It only takes a small amount of sodium—about the amount found in 1/4 teaspoon of salt—to meet our daily needs. Many people exceed this amount at every meal. It's not hard to go overboard eating salt; sodium occurs naturally in many foods and is added liberally to most processed foods. Fortunately, the taste for salty foods is one that is easy to curb. Retrain your taste buds to enjoy the more subtle and complex flavors of foods by replacing the salt shaker at the dining table with a variety of interesting herbal mixtures. Try toasted sesame seeds combined with oregano, basil, thyme, and freshly ground black pepper or experiment with the many herbal seasoning blends that are available at your natural foods store. I like using sea salt in cooking and don't believe that it's necessary for most people to eliminate it entirely from their diets. But I always slash the amount of salt suggested in recipes by at least half, and no one ever notices the difference. Cut back on salt, and you'll quickly notice how overly salty most commercially prepared foods are. The last time I bought a package of pretzels at the natural foods store, I had to brush the salt off of them to make them edible!

Cleansing Foods for the Kidneys

During a detoxification program, you can help your kidneys in their job of purification by increasing your intake of fluids. The kidneys need sufficient fluids flowing through them to efficiently flush toxins from the body. Drinking extra water has a natural, gentle diuretic effect. Strive for 6 to 8 glasses of pure water daily—either filtered water or spring water. Add a squeeze of fresh lemon or lime juice to add interest to plain water, or make a simple herbal tea to stimulate your desire to drink more fluids. Try peppermint, fennel seed, chamomile, or linden flower for pleasant tasting herbal beverages.

Many vegetables and fruits have natural diuretic properties and also stimulate kidney cleansing. A day of fasting on fresh juices can be very beneficial for purifying the kidneys and will improve their ability to cleanse the blood. To make a simple kidney cleansing tonic, juice carrots with beets, parsley, and cucumber. Add fresh ginger juice or a squeeze of fresh lemon or lime if desired. Sip an 8-ounce glass of fresh juice every couple of hours throughout the day, for a total of 6 glasses. In between, drink purified water and herbal teas. Plan to fast when you can rest and relax and be as free of responsibilities as possible.

In the spring, take advantage of the natural kidney cleansing benefits of fresh asparagus, and enjoy eating a portion of this delightful vegetable daily. Asparagus has natural diuretic properties and is a traditional tonic for purifying the kidneys. During the hot summer months, indulge frequently in fresh ripe watermelon. The juicy sweet melon is an excellent kidney cleanser. Be sure to eat watermelon on an empty stomach, either 30 minutes before a meal or 2 hours after. For many people, melons are difficult to digest when eaten with other foods, and tend to produce gas and intestinal discomfort.

KIDNEY CLEANSING FOODS AND JUICES

Asparagus

Parsley

Cucumber

Beets

Dandelion greens

Watercress

Cranberries

Grapes

Watermelon

Stimulate Kidney Function with Ginger Compresses

Ginger compresses can be used once or twice a week during a cleansing program to bring concentrated circulation to the kidneys and to stimulate the release of toxins. To prepare a ginger compress, grate a handful of ginger, place it in a piece of cheesecloth, twist to make a ball, and tie with a piece of string. Fill a large pot with 1 gallon of water, squeeze the ginger juice into the water, and drop the ball of ginger into the water. Cover the pot and heat the water, but don't boil it. Turn off the heat. Make a compress by folding a cotton handtowel in half lengthwise. Dip the towel into the hot ginger water, keeping the ends dry to prevent burning your fingers. Wring the compress out and place it over the kidneys, being careful to not burn the skin. You might need to let the compress cool for a few seconds before it can be placed onto the skin. Cover the compress with a dry towel to retain the heat. When the hot towel cools to body temperature, replace it with a fresh, hot compress. Continue placing hot compresses over the kidney area until the skin turns bright red, which usually takes about 15 to 20 minutes.

Kidney Purifying Herbal Tea

Many herbs have diuretic properties and promote the release of excess fluids from the body while stimulating kidney cleansing. Some, such as marshmallow root, have mucilagenous properties, and are traditionally used to soothe irritated mucous membranes. Try the following gentle kidney tea while cleansing, but avoid drinking it or any other diuretic tea before going to bed, for obvious reasons.

Gentle Diuretic Tea

1 teaspoon dandelion leaf

1 teaspoon marshmallow root

1 cup water

Pour boiling water over herbal mixture and cover. Let steep until cool. Strain, sweeten if desired, and drink at room temperature.

HERBS FOR THE KIDNEYS

Diuretic Herbs:

Dandelion leaf

Nettle

Marshmallow root

Cornsilk

Cleavers

Parsley

Antiseptic Diuretics:

Uva ursi

Juniper berry

Yarrow

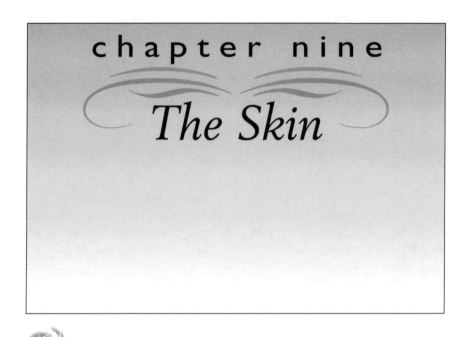

chapter nine

The Skin

Your Body's Master Detoxifier

Much more than just an external covering to hold your body together, your skin is the largest organ of your body, and is your physical connection to the outer world. Your sensations of touch, hot, cold, pain, and pressure are all conveyed through exquisitely sensitive nerve endings in the skin. The skin is composed of two layers, a thin outer layer, or *epidermis*, which consists of sheets of cells that become progressively flatter near the surface of the body, and the inner layer, or *dermis*, which is made up of a complex tangle of fibrous and elastic tissue that contains the blood vessels, nerves, hair follicles, and sweat glands.

A primary function of the skin is to help to maintain a constant body temperature. When you get too hot, your skin cools you down by perspiring. As droplets of sweat evaporate from the surface of your skin, your body temperature drops. Sweating also plays an important role in detoxification because toxins—including heavy metals, drugs, pesticides, and other environmental pollutants—are eliminated through perspiration. For this reason, the skin is sometimes referred to as the "third kidney." Approximately twenty-five percent of the body's waste products are excreted through the skin. If the skin is not efficiently expelling wastes, the other organs of elimination are burdened with excess toxins. Conversely, if the large intestine, kidneys, or liver are not adequately detoxifying and disposing of wastes, the burden falls to the skin. Acne, boils, skin rashes, and other eruptions are signals that something is amiss in the internal workings of the body's detoxification system. Look to your skin as a mirror for what is occuring inside of your body. While applying salves and other medicinal skin preparations can help to alleviate skin problems, the key to healthy skin requires attending to all of the organs of detoxification.

Andrea, 32, had suffered from periodic outbreaks of acne since she was a teenager. She attended my class in detoxification and enthusiastically started on a cleansing program. She ate an abundance of fresh vegetables and fruits and other high-fiber foods to cleanse her intestinal tract and purify her lymphatic system, drank 2 quarts of pure water and herbal teas daily to detoxify her kidneys and liver, and enjoyed daily herbal facials. Andrea was delighted to find that her skin began to clear up dramatically after only 2 weeks of following the cleansing program.

SYMPTOMS OF POOR SKIN FUNCTION

Acne

Clogged pores

Excessively oily skin

Excessively dry skin

Skin rashes

Eczema

Slow wound healing

Protecting Your Skin

In addition to cooling and detoxifying the body, the skin acts as the first line of defense against harmful microorganisms. Friendly bacteria that live on the surface of the skin prevent infiltration by bacteria, viruses, fungi, and parasites. To keep the skin healthy, remember that it is a vital, living organ and adopt the practice of not putting anything onto your skin that you wouldn't put into your mouth. Your skin absorbs into your bloodstream approximately 60 percent of whatever you apply to it, so you are essentially eating your bodycare products. In addition, antiperspirants and other chemicals applied to the skin kill off friendly skin bacteria, leaving you vulnerable to attack by unfriendly microorganisms.

A wide variety of excellent natural bodycare products are available at natural foods stores or by mail-order. Cultivate the habit of reading labels, and choose only the purest bodycare products, made from good quality vegetable oils, herbs, essential oils, and other natural ingredients. It's also easy, fun, and inexpensive to make your own bodycare products. See the Resource section for references that provide step-by-step instructions. In addition to using only natural bodycare products, choose natural fibers such as cotton, silk, linen, and wool for your clothing and bedding. Avoid synthetic fabrics, which inhibit perspiration and can irritate the skin.

Foods for Healthy Skin

Fresh vegetables and fruits, whole grains, lean proteins, good quality fats and oils, and plenty of pure water are the basics for good skin health. These foods promote the healthy functioning of the internal organs, which is reflected in the condition of the skin. High-fiber foods move wastes quickly through the large intestine, plenty of water flushes toxins out of the body through the kidneys, and an abundance of fresh, leafy green vegetables keeps the liver working efficiently to detoxify the bloodstream. Glowing, smooth, and blemish-free skin is an indication that all is well internally.

Dry, dull, and flaking skin often points to a deficiency of essential fatty acids in the diet. I've seen many people with dry skin and hair caused by their adherence to an excessively low-fat diet. Fat is a necessary nutrient. Instead of cutting fat out of your diet, focus on eating healthy fats, such as extra-virgin olive oil, almonds, avocados, pumpkin seeds, and sesame seeds. In addition, consider including sources of *omega-3* and *gamma-linolenic (GLA) essential fatty acids* in your diet. These special nutrients help to keep the skin supple and well-lubricated, and have many other whole-body health benefits as well. For more information on essential fatty acids, see Chapter 13.

Omega-3 oils are abundant in oily fish such as salmon, sardines, and mackerel. Approximately 3 servings per week (about 10 ounces total) is an ample amount for most people. Flaxseeds are also an excellent source of omega-3 fatty acids, and can be consumed either in the seed form or as an oil. Flax oil quickly becomes rancid and must be protected from heat and light. Buy it in small quantities in opaque containers, keep it refrigerated, do not cook with it, and use it within 6 weeks of opening the bottle. Flax oil has a relatively mild taste, and can be used on salads, baked potatoes, or pasta. If you choose to eat flaxseeds, they must be ground instead of eaten whole—otherwise, they will pass through your intestinal tract undigested. I have an electric coffee grinder that I reserve for grinding flaxseeds, and within seconds, it makes fresh flax meal. Flaxseeds have a mild, nutty flavor and are delicious when added to oatmeal or another cooked cereal just before serving. Ground flaxseeds can also be whipped into a healthy beverage in the blender with fruit juice, soy milk, or almond milk, along with bananas or other fresh fruit. Flaxseeds have mucilagenous properties and become gel-like when added to liquid, so plan to consume your beverage immediately after preparing it. Eat 1 to 4 tablespoons of freshly ground flaxseeds daily or 1 to 2 tablespoons of flax oil.

HEALTHY FATS FOR THE SKIN

Extra virgin olive oil

Sesame seeds

Pumpkin seeds

Walnuts

Almonds

Sunflower seeds

Avocados

Omega-3 fatty acids:

Oily fish (salmon, sardines)

Flaxseeds and flax oil

Gamma-linolenic acid:

Evening primrose oil

Black currant oil

Borage oil

Gamma-linolenic acid (GLA) is helpful for treating dry skin and hair, eczema, and other skin disorders. While GLA can be synthesized from the linoleic acid found in most nuts, seeds, and grains, in reality, many people suffer from a deficiency of this essential fatty acid. Factors that interfere with GLA conversion include consumption of *trans-fatty acids* (found in polyunsaturated oils and hydrogenated oils) and saturated fats, alcohol and tobacco, nutrient deficiencies, and aging. Evening primrose oil, black currant seed oil, and borage oil are rich sources of GLA and are available as supplements. Take enough capsules to equal approximately 240 milligrams of GLA daily.

Eliminate Toxins with Saunas

While drinking plenty of pure water will help to keep your skin hydrated and facilitate the release of toxins, you can also take advantage of the purifying benefits of water externally through the use of saunas, steams, and special cleansing baths. A daily bath or shower removes surface perspiration and toxins. But you don't want to dry out your skin or upset the natural protective acid mantle. Use gentle vegetable oil soaps and lather up only where you absolutely need to. A thorough scrubbing with warm water and a loofah or rough washcloth is all you need over most of your body to remove dry skin cells and refresh your skin. Be sure to install a water filter on your shower if your tap water is chlorinated. Your skin and your hair will be much softer and you won't be absorbing chlorine, which is a potent toxin.

Wet saunas and steam baths are a wonderful method of purification. The combination of heat and steam stimulates circulation and opens the pores, helping the skin to expel toxins. Saunas are so effective at promoting cleansing that they are an integral part of medical detoxification programs for people who have been exposed to highly toxic chemicals. Before using a sauna or steam bath, apply olive oil liberally to your entire body with gentle massage strokes. For a fragrant massage oil, combine 30 drops of sandalwood or lavender essential oil with 2 ounces of extra virgin olive oil. According to Ayurvedic medicine, the oil penetrates the skin and helps to expel toxins from the body tissues. I've found that applying oil before a sauna definitely promotes increased perspiration and also leaves my skin feeling soft and well-moisturized.

Regular saunas taken once a week can help to keep you in optimal health. During a cleansing program, use saunas or steam baths 2 or 3 times a week if possible. A wet sauna or steam is best and easiest on the body. If you only have a dry sauna available, use a mister bottle to spray your body every couple of minutes. Set the temperature at a moderate setting, somewhere between 140 and 160 degrees. A moderately hot sauna that you can remain in comfortably for 10 or 15 minutes at a time promotes the release of toxins much more effectively than a scalding hot sauna that you can only tolerate for a few minutes. Three 10-minute sessions or 2, 15-minute sessions provides excellent detoxification benefits. In between, rinse off with a tepid shower. Be sure to keep a towel covering your head while in the sauna to prevent overheating. Drink plenty of fluids before, during, and after your sauna to stimulate the excretion of toxins and to keep the body well-hydrated. If at any time you experience dizziness or nausea, discontinue the sauna. Finish up your sauna or steam session with a cool shower.

If you are pregnant, or have high blood pressure or cardiovascular disease, do not use saunas or steam baths or other hot baths without consulting your health care practitioner.

Epsom salts baths are also helpful for promoting deep cleansing of toxins through the skin. For a simple detoxifying bath, add 2 cups of Epsom salts to a bathtub of hot water. Soak for 20 minutes, sponging your face with a cool cloth while in the tub. To intensify the purifying benefits of the bath, drink a cleansing herbal tea made from herbs that promote perspiration. Drink 1 cup before entering the bath and another cup while soaking in the tub. For a variety of purifying bath treatments, see Chapter 15.

Cleansing Herbal Tea

1 teaspoon yarrow flowers

1 teaspoon peppermint leaves

1 teaspoon fennel seeds

2 cups filtered water

Simmer the fennel seeds in 2 cups of water in a covered pot for 5 minutes. Turn off the heat, add the yarrow and peppermint, cover the pot, and let steep for 10 minutes. Strain, and drink hot.

Salt Scrub for Glowing Skin

A sea salt scrub with essential oils removes the top layer of dead skin cells and improves skin function and texture. Mix 1 tablespoon of olive or almond oil with 1/2 cup of fine sea salt and 10 drops of sandlewood or lavender essential oil. The oil in this scrub makes the tub dangerously slick, so be sure to use a rubber tub mat to keep from slipping. Stand in the shower and rinse your body with warm water. Scoop up a small handful of the salt and oil mixture and rub it gently into your skin, beginning with your legs and working up your body. Massage with a circular motion, avoiding your genitals and face and any areas with broken skin. After you have covered your entire body with the scrub, rinse thoroughly with warm water. This treatment can be used once a week to keep your skin smooth and glowing.

Herbs for the Skin

Many herbs for the skin are traditionally called "blood cleansers," which refers to their ability to improve the function of the liver, large intestine, and kidneys in eliminating wastes. In addition, herbs with diaphoretic properties act directly on the skin to increase surface blood flow and to promote perspiration, thus helping the skin to excrete toxins more efficiently.

HERBS FOR THE SKIN

Blood Cleansers:

Sarsaparilla

Yellow dock

Burdock

Oregon grape

Red clover

Nettle

Diaphoretics:

Yarrow

Peppermint

Elder flower

Ginger

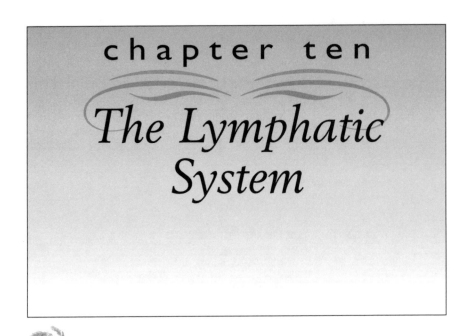

chapter ten

The Lymphatic System

Your Body's Master Blood Cleanser

The lymphatic system plays an integral part in detoxification. It transports lymph, a clear, colorless fluid that bathes and purifies all of the cells of your body. The lymphatic system runs parallel to the circulatory system and is composed of a network of porous lymphatic vessels that are similar to arteries, as well as hundreds of lymph nodes that are scattered throughout the body. Lymph passes into and out of the bloodstream through permeable membranes, bringing nutrients to the cells and carrying away waste products. The waste materials transported out of the cells are filtered through lymph nodes, which are clustered primarily in the armpits, neck, groin, abdomen, and chest. The *tonsils, adenoids, appendix, spleen,* and *Peyer's patches* in the small intestine are also part of the lymphatic system. The tonsils, adenoids, appendix, and spleen have erroneously been considered as disposable by the medical profession, when in fact they play an essential role in detoxification. Along with the lymph nodes, these organs filter toxins from the lymph, and destroy harmful microorganisms and cellular wastes such as worn-out blood cells.

The lymphatic system plays a critical role in your body's immune functioning. Within the lymph nodes, white blood cells such as *lymphocytes* and *macrophages* attack and consume troublemaking microorganisms. During an infection, the lymph nodes closest to the affected area swell to contain the toxins. You've most likely experienced tender, swollen lymph nodes under your jaw when you've had a sore throat. The swollen nodes indicate that the lymph system is working hard to overpower the invading microorganisms. When the infection has run its course, the lymph nodes return to their normal state, which is about the size of a small pea.

Although the lymphatic system does have some similarities to the circulatory system, it does not have the luxury of its own private pump, as does the circulatory system. The heart regularly pumps blood throughout the arteries, but the lymphatic system relies on external pressure, such as exercise, breathing, and massage, to move the lymph. Consequently, many people suffer from poor lymphatic function. When the lymph is not flowing freely, stagnation occurs, wastes back up in the cells, and infections are more likely to gain a foothold.

If you have swollen lymph nodes that occur without evidence of an infection, or that persist after an infection has run its course, consult your health care practitioner.

SYMPTOMS OF POOR LYMPHATIC FUNCTION

Swollen lymph nodes

Frequent infections

Tender lymph nodes

Hardened lymph nodes

Cellulite

Lymphatic-Purifying Diet

A simple cleansing diet helps to purify the lymphatic system. Certain foods tend to produce an excess of waste products that thicken lymphatic fluids. The thicker the lymph, the more difficulty it has in cleansing the cells. To promote healthy lymph, avoid fatty foods, dairy products, red meat, processed and refined foods, and sugars. The most cleansing foods for the lymphatic system are fresh vegetables and fruits. Try to make vegetables and fruits approximately 50 percent of your daily food intake. I keep this uncomplicated by making sure that about half of the food on my plate at lunch and dinner consists of vegetables. In between meals, I snack on fresh fruits. Fresh vegetables and fruits are rich in vitamins, minerals, and contain the unquantifiable vibrant life energy of the plant. If you make only one change in your dietary habits, make it this. Within a few days of increasing your intake of fresh vegetables and fruits, you will notice a significant difference in your level of well-being.

Carolyn was dismayed to find that her thighs and buttocks were riddled with cellulite, even after losing 20 pounds. She attended one of my cleansing programs, and immediately made the connection between her sedentary lifestyle, poor dietary habits, and cellulite. She began eating an abundance of fresh vegetables and fruits, started walking and doing yoga stretches daily, and took saunas twice a week. She also performed vigorous dry body brushing and lymphatic massage daily. Two months later, she reported a dramatic decrease in cellulite, along with an abundance of vitality!

DIET FOR LYMPHATIC HEALTH

Avoid:

Dairy products

Red meat

Fatty foods

Refined foods

Processed sugars

Emphasize:

Fresh vegetables

Fresh fruits

Exercise for a Healthy Lymphatic System

Because the lymph system has no pump, it relies on you to help keep lymph flowing. Exercise has many whole body benefits, and it is the primary way of moving lymph throughout the body. If you are sedentary, your lymph is also sluggish, which contributes to a general feeling of lethargy. When you exercise, the contraction of your muscles and the increase in your rate and depth of breathing stimulates the smooth flow of lymph. Any activity that gets you moving is beneficial, so choose an exercise that you enjoy—you'll be more likely to stick with it. Walking, dancing, and swimming are all excellent for stimulating lymph flow. The best activities are those that have rhythmical movements and involve as much of your body as possible. Set a goal of at least 30 minutes of vigorous exercise daily. Studies have shown that people who engage in regular moderate exercise have stronger immune systems and are less likely to come down with colds and flus. Each time you exercise, you are helping your body to detoxify by stimulating lymphatic flow, which cleanses your cells.

Enhance Lymphatic Flow with Massage

Don't substitute massage for exercise, but do consider including massage as a regular part of your health enhancement program. A whole body massage is excellent for stimulating lymphatic flow. The lymphatic system is close to the surface of the body, and massage manually pushes the lymph through the lymph channels. Treat yourself to a professional massage at least once a month, or more often if possible. While cleansing, schedule a massage once or even twice a week. Consider trading massages with your partner or a friend. Massage techniques are easy to learn and there are excellent books and videos available that take you step-by-step through a full body massage. See the Resource section for massage book and video recommendations.

You can also use simple self-massage techniques at home every day that will improve lymphatic function. A dry brush massage before showering enhances the flow of lymph and benefits the skin by removing dry, dead skin cells. To perform a dry brush massage, you'll need a natural bristle body brush. I like using a brush with a handle, so that I can easily brush my shoulders and back. Buy a brush with bristles that will comfortably stimulate your skin without scratching it. Beginning with your feet, brush with long strokes up your calves and your thighs. Brush vigorously, but be careful to not irritate your skin. Always brush in the direction of your heart, which is the natural direction of lymphatic flow. Brush up your hips, lower back, and abdomen, and then up your arms and across your shoulders and back. Brush gently across your chest, and avoid your face and any areas with broken or irritated skin.

My favorite self-massage technique is a hot towel scrub, which invigorates lymphatic flow and is a wonderful way to begin the day or to use just before going to bed at night. Fill a basin with very hot water, and add 5 drops of lavender essential oil. Stir the oil into the water. Dip a cotton terry washcloth into the water and wring it out, being careful not to burn yourself. Beginning with one foot, vigorously rub until it turns rosy with increased circulation. Dip your washcloth into the hot water again and wring it out, and vigorously rub your calf. Repeat the process, working up your thigh, and then begin on the opposite foot and leg. Massage always toward your heart, in the direction of lymphatic flow. Continue rubbing the hot washcloth over your entire body except for your face, scrubbing briskly to stimulate circulation and lymphatic flow. A hot towel scrub takes no more than 5 or 10 minutes, and will leave you feeling refreshed and cleansed. I've made a habit of using this simple treatment before retiring for the night, and it always ensures a deep, restful, and healing sleep.

Footbath to Increase Lymph Circulation

Alternating hot and cold footbaths is another pleasurable method for increasing lymphatic flow. Gravity naturally pulls lymph down to your feet, and the stimulating effects of hot and cold water help to move stagnant lymph. You'll need two buckets, each one large enough to hold both of your feet. Fill one bucket with water as hot as you can tolerate, and fill the other with cold water. The water should be deep enough to cover your feet to above your ankles. For additional stimulating and detoxifying benefits, mix 5 drops each of rosemary and juniper essential oils in 1 teaspoon of witch hazel and add to the bucket of hot water. Sit in a comfortable chair, place your feet in the bucket of hot water, and relax for 3 minutes. Immediately plunge your feet into the bucket of cold water for 30 seconds. Repeat this sequence 3 times, ending with the cold water plunge. Pat your feet dry, and finish with long, sweeping massage strokes with the palms of your hands up your calves and thighs to draw the lymph upward.

Lymph-Purifying Herbal Tea

Herbs that improve lymphatic function are those with specific immune-enhancing properties, such as echinacea and goldenseal, and others which are traditionally used as lymphatic cleansers, such as red clover and cleavers. Lymph cleansing herbs are helpful when included as part of a detoxification program to stimulate cell purification. In addition, potent antimicrobial herbs such as echinacea and goldenseal are especially helpful for boosting lymphatic function at any time when the body is battling an infection. If it's spring, you can probably find the herbs for this tea in your own backyard. Consult a good herbal identification book if you are not familiar with the plants.

Gentle Lymph-Cleansing Herbal Tea

2 tablespoons fresh red clover blossoms
(or 2 teaspoons dried)
2 tablespoons fresh cleavers, aerial parts
(or 2 teaspoons dried)
2 cups filtered or spring water
Pour boiling water over the herbs, cover, and let steep for 15 minutes. Strain, and drink.

HERBS FOR THE LYMPHATIC SYSTEM

Cleavers

Mullein

Red clover

Prickly ash

Echinacea

Goldenseal

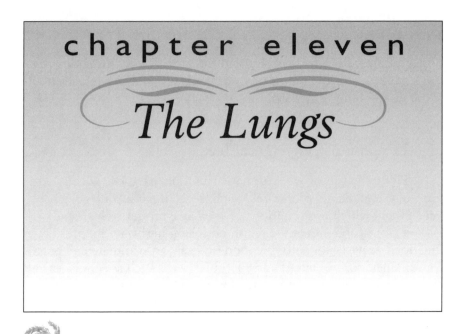

chapter eleven

The Lungs

Your Body's Master Oxygenator

Somewhere between 10 and 20 times a minute, your lungs expand and contract, bringing life-giving oxygen to all of the cells of your body, and expelling poisonous carbon dioxide wastes. The lungs supply us with the most essential nutrient of all, for while you can live for days without food or water, you can survive for only a matter of minutes without oxygen. Oxygen is necessary for virtually every biochemical process that takes place in the body.

The process of oxygenating the cells begins when air is inhaled through the nostrils, down the *trachea* (commonly called the windpipe), and into the lungs. Filling most of the chest cavity, the lungs are spongelike organs that work in harmony with the cardiovascular system to supply the body with oxygen. Blood that has circulated through the body returns to the heart through the veins, where it is pumped through the right side of the heart and into the lungs via the *pulmonary arteries*. Within the lungs, these arteries branch out much like a tree. Small blood vessels at the tips of the branches are surrounded by tiny air sacs called *alveoli* that transfer fresh oxygen to the blood and remove carbon dioxide. The cleansed blood with its fresh supply of oxygen then flows back to the heart, where it is pumped from the left side throughout the body.

In their role of detoxification, the lungs expel toxic carbon dioxide gas from the body. Carbon dioxide is a waste product of normal body processes, and is produced by cells when nutrients such as glucose are broken down. Many people breathe shallowly, using only a small amount of their lung capacity. This leaves residues of carbon dioxide in the bloodstream and leads to symptoms of toxicity such as fatigue. By paying conscious attention to your patterns of breathing, you can create dramatic changes in your health. Learning to breathe fully is one of the most powerful tools you have for cleansing your body.

Along with poor breathing patterns, environmental toxins such as smog, exhaust fumes, industrial pollutants, smoke, and airborne allergens all contribute to impaired lung function. The lungs thrive on fresh, clean air. Treat your lungs as often as possible to places where the air is pure; the ocean, mountains, running streams and rivers, and forests are sources of oxygen-rich air. If you're in the city, search out parks and arboretums and other places where trees and shrubs are abundant.

If you suffer from chronic bronchitis, unexplained coughing, chest pain, or other symptoms of respiratory distress, consult your health care practitioner.

SYMPTOMS OF POOR LUNG FUNCTION

Shallow breathing

Fatigue

Bronchitis

Chronic coughs

Congestion

Diet for a Healthy Respiratory System

During a detoxification program, you can help to cleanse your lungs by reducing your intake of foods which tend to promote the formation of excess mucus. Mucus is necessary in the body. It lubricates mucous membranes and also helps the body to eliminate wastes. But an excess of mucus can lead to congestion, which is often most apparent in the respiratory system. A diet low in mucus-promoting foods is especially helpful in cases of chronic congestion, such as sinusitis and bronchitis, and for alleviating respiratory allergies.

The primary foods which contribute to congestion are dairy products, flour products, refined foods, and sugars. Wheat in any form seems to be especially congesting, and for some people, all gluten-containing grains (wheat, oats, barley, and rye) are best avoided. Substitute other grains such as rice, buckwheat, millet, and quinoa. Fresh vegetables and fruits are low in mucus-forming activity and help to cleanse the body. Simply sipping hot water with lemon can help to reduce mucus congestion and cleanse accumulation from the respiratory tract.

CONGESTING FOODS

Dairy products

Refined foods

Sugar

Flour products

Wheat, oats, barley, rye

Exercise for Healthy Lungs

Vigorous exercise increases the body's demand for oxygen, which encourages you to breathe more deeply and enhances the rate at which the body eliminates carbon dioxide. That's why a brisk walk is so invigorating for your body and your mind; your cells are receiving extra oxygen and at the same time getting rid of the toxic wastes that contribute to fatigue. Because exercise makes you breathe more deeply, the capacity of the lungs to take in oxygen and eliminate carbon dioxide is improved. If the lungs are not regularly used to their full capacity, they begin to lose their elasticity. Any brisk, vigorous exercise that increases your rate of breathing will improve your lung capacity and helps your lungs to detoxify your bloodstream. Brisk walking, dancing, gardening, hiking, bicycling, and swimming are all excellent choices. Obviously, avoid exercising in polluted areas. I am always dismayed to see people jogging alongside highways, breathing in deeply the exhaust fumes and road dust. Search out places to exercise that have fresh, clean air. Also consider the time of day that you exercise; the air often seems to be most pure early in the morning.

Oxygenate Your Body with Deep-Breathing Exercises

By taking a few minutes daily to focus specifically on your breathing, you can increase your lung capacity and the ability of your lungs to purify your body. Deep-breathing exercises immediately promote a feeling of relaxation and well-being, and with regular practice, will help to increase your energy, promote clear thinking, and improve the quality of your sleep. The ancient art of yoga is an excellent method for increasing your awareness of your breathing patterns, and will stretch and rejuvenate your entire body while enhancing your control of your breath. See Chapter 14 for specific directions for practicing healing yoga postures.

Simple breathing exercises that you can do anywhere, anytime are invaluable for improving your breathing and your overall health. The following exercise will help you to become aware of how to breathe fully. It may feel awkward at first, especially if you are in the habit of breathing shallowly.

Sit or lie in a comfortable position, and place your hands on your belly. Inhale through your nose, and allow the breath to flow down into your abdomen. Your abdomen should expand as you inhale. As you continue to inhale, allow the breath to flow upward into your lungs, and your chest to expand. Hold for just a moment, and then let the air flow out of your body in the reverse order. As you exhale, feel the breath first flow out of the top portion of your lungs as your chest falls. Completely exhale by pulling your abdomen in toward your spine to expel all the air from your lungs. Pause for a moment, and repeat. Continue breathing in this way for a few minutes. Be gentle, and don't force the breath. It takes time to learn how to breathe fully. Another good exercise for expanding the capacity of the lungs is to practice blowing up a balloon several times a day. For more suggestions on breathing exercises to promote cleansing and rejuvenation, see Chapter 16.

Soothing Herbal Inhalation

An herbal steam inhalation is an excellent method for loosening congestion and cleansing the lungs. Steam inhalations are particularly helpful for relieving chronic sinusitis, respiratory congestion, bronchitis, and colds and flus, and can be used as often as desired for treating these conditions. The warm steam eases congested breathing, and the volatile essential oils from the herbs release their healing vapors into the steam and help to cleanse the lungs while promoting the expulsion of mucus. Adding antimicrobial herbs such as thyme, eucalyptus, or peppermint to an herbal steam helps to fight infection in the lungs.

To make an herbal steam inhalation, place 1 1/2 quarts of water in a large pot with 2 tablespoons each of dried thyme and peppermint. Bring the water to a boil over medium heat, cover, and turn off the heat. Allow the herbs to steep for 10 minutes. Place the pot on a table, remove the lid, and cover your head and the pot of steaming herbs with a large towel. Breathe in the steam, taking care not to burn yourself. Stay under the towel tent for 15 minutes, lifting the towel as necessary to regulate the steam.

Mustard Plaster to Relieve Lung Congestion

A stimulating mustard plaster is excellent for breaking up deep lung congestion and helping the lungs to expel mucus. This plaster is helpful for treating chronic bronchitis, colds, flus, and other respiratory problems, and can be applied either to the chest or to the upper back. To make the plaster, mix 2 tablespoons of powdered mustard and 4 tablespoons of flour with enough hot water to make a spreadable paste. Dip a thin cotton dish towel into hot water and wring it out. Spread the mustard paste onto the towel and fold the towel to make a flat pack, with the mustard paste on the inside of the pack. Place the pack directly on the chest or the upper back and cover the entire area with a thick towel. Leave the plaster in place for about 20 minutes, lifting a corner of the plaster every few minutes to make sure that the mustard is not burning the skin. A feeling of warmth and a healthy pink color indicates that the plaster is working, but if an uncomfortable burning sensation, redness, or irritation occurs, remove the plaster.

Herbal Tea for Healthy Lungs

Many herbs for the lungs have soothing, demulcent properties which help to heal the mucous membranes of the lungs. These soothing herbs act as tonics to improve lung health. Other herbs for the lungs have expectorant action, and help to loosen and eliminate excess mucus. The following tea is an excellent soothing tonic for the lungs.

Lung Tonic Tea

1 tablespoon licorice root

1 tablespoon mullein leaf

1 tablespoon marshmallow root

3 cups filtered or spring water

Simmer licorice root in water for 10 minutes. Remove from heat, add mullein leaf and marshmallow root and steep, covered, for 15 minutes. Strain, and drink warm, up to 3 cups a day.

HERBS FOR THE LUNGS

Demulcents:

Mullein

Licorice root

Flax seed

Marshmallow root

Fenugreek

Expectorants:

Thyme

Eucalyptus

Licorice root

Fenugreek

Mullein

PART THREE

CREATING
A CLEANSING
PROGRAM

chapter twelve

Herbs: Potent Allies for Cleansing and Rejuvenation

*H*erbs have been used for centuries for purification and rejuvenation, and the plants which stimulate and support the body's natural cleansing processes are highly valued in all traditional forms of natural medicine. Purifying herbs improve the circulation of blood and lymph, stimulate the elimination of toxins, and enhance the functioning of the liver, kidneys, intestines, lungs, lymphatic system, and skin. Helping the body to detoxify allows deep healing and rejuvenation to take place.

All of the herbs recommended here have a long history of safe use. Nonetheless, many do have powerful cleansing actions and should be used wisely. Always pay attention to how your body responds to the herbs you are using, and if you notice any unusual reactions or have any questions or concerns, stop using the herbs and consult your health care practitioner for advice. If you are pregnant or nursing, or if you have a serious health condition, use detoxifying herbs only under the guidance of your health care practitioner.

Seven Powerful Ways Herbs Promote Cleansing

Herbs work in a variety of ways to stimulate cleansing. Understanding the ways that these healing plants help to purify your body will demystify the process of detoxification and will

enable you to design a balanced cleansing program. When undertaking a detoxification program, it is essential to support all of your
body's pathways of cleansing. This prevents any one organ system
from being overburdened with toxins, and facilitates a deep level of
purification.

Hepatic Herbs

Hepatics are herbs that work specifically on the liver. Because
the liver is so critical to the process of detoxification, supporting the
liver during a cleansing program is essential. I always include hepatic herbs as a central part of any detoxification plan. Hepatic herbs
are primarily herbs with a bitter flavor, such as dandelion root, gentian root, Oregon grape root, and yellow dock root. The bitter quality of these herbs stimulates bile flow, which naturally cleanses the
liver. Make a pot of liver-cleansing tea to drink daily during a detoxification program, or take a tincture of liver-cleansing herbs 3 to 4
times daily. If you suffer from poor digestive function, bitter herbs
can be taken on a regular basis in the form of a digestive bitters tonic
to encourage the secretion of digestive enzymes (see recipe on p.
126).

HEPATIC HERBS

Dandelion root

Burdock

Yellow dock

Oregon grape

Licorice

Barberry

Sarsaparilla

Gentian

Turmeric

Milk thistle

Some herbs for the liver have powerful restorative properties,
and are especially helpful for protecting the liver against the deluge

of toxins that threaten the well-being of this vital organ. Milk thistle seed is a specific restorative tonic for the liver. It has been found to stimulate healthy cell regeneration even when the liver has been severely damaged by toxic substances. And turmeric, the deep yellow spice that is the primary ingredient in curry powder, is a potent antioxidant that protects the liver from harmful toxins. I recommend taking liver-protective herbs on a regular basis to strengthen and heal the liver. Grind a couple of tablespoons of milk thistle seeds and sprinkle onto hot or cold cereals, and cultivate the habit of cooking with turmeric—it adds a beautiful golden hue to soups, curries, and sauces.

Diuretic Herbs

Diuretic herbs work specifically on the kidneys and urinary tract to stimulate increased urination. They help the body to eliminate excess water and at the same time cleanse the urinary tract. Examples of diuretic herbs include dandelion leaf, which probably grows in your backyard, and the common kitchen herb, parsley. Dandelion has been found to be as effective as commonly prescribed pharmaceutical diuretics, but without the harmful side effects. Synthetic diuretics deplete the body of potassium and can cause serious problems such as muscle weakness and cardiac arrythmias. In the infinite wisdom of nature, both dandelion leaf and parsley are rich in potassium, which makes them safe diuretics.

Drinking a couple of cups of gentle diuretic tea daily during a cleansing program is helpful for flushing the kidneys and urinary tract. Women who suffer from premenstrual water retention often obtain significant relief by drinking 3 to 4 cups of a cleansing diuretic tea in the week to 10 days preceeding menstruation. However, even when using herbal diuretics, be sure to eat foods that are naturally rich sources of potassium, such as leafy green vegetables, potatoes, citrus fruits, and apples.

Juniper berries and uva ursi have strong antimicrobial action in addition to their diuretic properties, which makes them an excellent choice for treating urinary tract infections. Drinking 2 quarts of juniper berry and uva ursi tea throughout the day at the first sign of a bladder infection (increased frequency of urination or a burning or stinging sensation while urinating) cleanses the bladder and will usually abort the infection. Juniper berries contain potent stimulating essential oils that can be irritating to the kidneys, and should not be used during pregnancy or if there is a history of kidney disease.

DIURETIC HERBS

Marshmallow root

Nettle

Cleavers

Corn silk

Burdock

Dandelion leaf

Parsley

Yarrow

Uva ursi

Juniper berries

Laxative Herbs

Laxative herbs are those which help to facilitate bowel movements. The most gentle are the fiber laxatives such as psyllium husks and flax seeds, which promote intestinal function by creating large, soft stools. Others, such as yellow dock and dandelion root, encourage the flow of bile, which has a natural laxative effect. Stronger laxative herbs (also called *purgatives*), such as cascara sagrada and senna, work directly on the colon by stimulating peristalsis, the contractions which move waste products through the large intestine. Herbs with purgative action should be combined with aromatic herbs such as ginger or fennel seeds to relieve possible intestinal cramping.

I recommend taking a fiber laxative daily during a cleansing program as an "intestinal broom" to help move toxins more rapidly through the intestinal tract and out of the body. Fiber laxatives are safe and can be taken on a regular basis if you suffer from sluggish intestinal function. Take 1 to 2 teaspoons of powdered psyllium husks or 1 to 2 tablespoons of soaked or ground flax seeds daily. Be sure to drink plenty of water when taking fiber laxatives. Psyllium and flax both absorb water, which causes them to swell and creates bulk in the intestinal tract. Not drinking enough water can create constipation instead of curing it.

Gentle laxatives such as yellow dock, dandelion root, and licorice root can also be taken daily during a cleansing program to further encourage colon cleansing. In addition to their laxative properties, these herbs are hepatics, and I often include one or more in a cleansing tea formula to improve both liver and intestinal function. If a stronger laxative is needed, I recommend cascara sagrada as a safe and effective choice. Take 1 dropperful of cascara sagrada tincture or 1 cup of cascara sagrada tea before bed, and repeat the dosage in the morning if necessary. While senna is included in many commercial laxatives and detoxification products, it has a much stronger action and can cause diarrhea and cramping. Senna should be used only if all else fails to relieve constipation. To prevent "lazy bowel" syndrome and laxative dependency, avoid using any stimulant laxatives on a regular basis.

LAXATIVE HERBS

Psyllium

Flax seeds

Licorice

Burdock

Dandelion root

Yellow dock

Cascara sagrada

Buckthorn

Senna

Diaphoretic Herbs

Diaphoretic herbs are those which stimulate perspiration by promoting increased circulation and dilating the capillaries at the surface of the skin. Approximately 25 percent of all toxins in the body are eliminated through the skin. By increasing perspiration, diaphoretics assist the skin in its role of purification.

During a cleansing program, I recommend drinking a cup or two of a diaphoretic tea before soaking in a detoxifying bath to intensify the effects of the bath. For best results, drink diaphoretic teas hot, to further stimulate sweating. All of the diaphoretic herbs suggested can also be made into strong teas and added to a hot bath to increase the elimination of toxins through the skin. To prepare an herbal tea for a bath, bring 2 quarts of water to a boil and add 1/2 cup of dried herb. Cover, and let steep until cool. Strain out the herb and add the liquid to a hot bath.

Diaphoretics are especially useful for treating colds and flus. Through encouraging perspiration, they support the body's efforts to eliminate the virus. I have many times stopped the onset of a cold or flu by soaking in a hot ginger or thyme bath and drinking hot ginger tea at the first sign of a sniffle or sore throat. If a cold or flu does take hold, a hot herbal bath and several cups of hot diaphoretic tea throughout the day is one of the best remedies for relieving chills and aches. If a cold or flu is accompanied by a fever, a combination of yarrow, peppermint, and elderflower tea works wonders to help naturally lower the fever through increasing perspiration. A tepid bath or sponge bath of the same tea is also helpful for relieving a fever.

DIAPHORETIC HERBS

Yarrow

Ginger

Peppermint

Thyme

Elder flowers

Lymphatic Herbs

Lymphatic herbs stimulate cleansing of the network of lymph vessels and glands throughout the body. The lymphatic vessels transport lymph, a colorless fluid that bathes and purifies all of the cells, tissues, and organs. Because the lymphatic system has no pump, it relies on external forces such as exercise or massage to move the lymph. Lymphatic herbs, such as cleavers, red clover, and prickly ash promote lymphatic flow and drainage. They can be taken as a tea or tincture to support lymph cleansing during a detoxification program.

When lymph flow stagnates, the body is more susceptible to infections. The lymph glands, located primarily in the neck, armpits, and groin and including the tonsils and spleen, are an essential component of the immune system. These trap foreign substances such as bacteria and produce infection-fighting white blood cells. Swollen and painful lymph glands indicate that your lymphatic system is fighting an infection. You can bolster your body's efforts with antimicrobial herbs such as echinacea and goldenseal. These safe and powerful herbs help to cleanse the lymphatic system and support the action of the lymph glands against harmful microorganisms. Because of the increased amount of toxins released during a detoxification program, I suggest taking echinacea tincture, 1 dropperful 3 times daily, for up to 2 weeks during a cleanse.

LYMPHATIC HERBS

Cleavers

Red clover

Prickly ash

Goldenseal

Echinacea

Expectorant Herbs

Expectorant herbs facilitate the removal of excessive mucus from the lungs and help to relieve congestion. While a thin coating of mucus is necessary to keep the mucous membranes healthy, too much mucus causes stagnation and creates a breeding ground for bacteria and viruses as well as interferes with healthy lung function.

Expectorants act on the entire respiratory system and are especially useful for supporting the body in overcoming colds, flus, and other respiratory illnesses. Some expectorant herbs, such as mullein and marshmallow, are mucilagenous—they have a slippery, soothing quality that helps to heal irritated bronchial tissues caused by allergies, air pollution, smoking, or bronchitis. These gentle herbs can be taken over a long period of time as tonics for the lungs. Other expectorants, such as thyme and eucalyptus, have potent antimicrobial action and help to cleanse the lungs of harmful microorganisms. They are especially useful for treating colds, flus, and other infections. Thyme and eucalyptus are also excellent to use in steam inhalations for relieving lung congestion. The potent volatile oils are released in the steam and when inhaled into the lungs, loosen excess mucus and provide direct antimicrobial action. To make a steam inhalation, bring 1 1/2 quarts of water to a boil, turn off the heat, and add 4 to 6 tablespoons of dried herb. Cover, and let steep for 10 minutes. Remove the lid, make a towel tent over the pot and your head, and inhale the steam for 10 minutes. Be careful not to scald yourself; lift the towel as necessary to regulate the steam.

EXPECTORANT HERBS

Licorice

Mullein

Marshmallow

Fenugreek

Fennel

Thyme

Eucalyptus

Peppermint

Antimicrobial Herbs

Antimicrobial herbs are those which have direct action against bacteria, viruses, fungi, and other microorganisms. They are especially useful for supporting cleansing during an infection such as a cold or flu or for overcoming a chronic condition such as *Candida albicans* overgrowth. Including antimicrobial herbs as part of a detoxification program is helpful for purifying the blood and lymphatic system, as well as assisting the body to eliminate unfriendly microorganisms that may be residing elsewhere in the body.

Eating 1 or 2 cloves of garlic daily is beneficial during a cleansing program. To obtain the antimicrobial properties, garlic must be eaten raw and either crushed or chopped. Try adding it to salad dressings, pasta, or soups just before serving. I also suggest taking 1 dropperful of echinacea tincture 3 times a day during a detoxification program. If your immunity is low and you tend to get every cold and flu that goes around, you might find it helpful to take echinacea for a couple of months to strengthen your immunity. When using echinacea for more than 2 weeks, take 1 week off for every 2 weeks that you take the herb. Echinacea is completely safe, but may work most effectively if it is not used continuously.

ANTIMICROBIAL HERBS

Echinacea

Goldenseal

Garlic

Thyme

Eucalyptus

Yarrow

Creating Herbal Cleansing Formulas

Guidelines for Choosing and Storing Herbs

Dried Herbs

- Choose herbs that are brightly colored and fragrant; this will ensure more potent herbal preparations. Whenever possible, purchase organically grown herbs.
- Store each herb individually in a tightly covered glass container. Pint or quart-size canning jars are ideal.
- Heat and light destroy the healing properties of herbs. Store your herbs in a cool, dark, dry place, such as a cabinet, pantry, or closet.
- When properly stored, the dried leaves and flowers of herbs will retain their medicinal properties for approximately 1 year. Most roots and barks will retain their healing properties for up to 2 years. In general, if an herb has kept its color and fragrance, it has retained its healing essence.

Herbal Tinctures

- ✑ Herbal tinctures are concentrated extracts made by steeping an herb in alcohol (such as grain alcohol or vodka) or vegetable glycerin. Occasionally, tinctures are made with apple cider vinegar. Alcohol best extracts the full range of medicinal properties of the herb and also acts as a preservative. Glycerin and apple cider vinegar are less effective at extracting the healing constituents of the plant, but are useful options for people who wish to avoid alcohol.

- ✑ You can evaporate off most of the alcohol from a tincture by placing the tincture dosage in a cup and pouring 1/4 cup of boiling water over it. Allow the water to cool for several minutes before drinking.

- ✑ Tinctures should be stored in a cool, dark, dry place. If stored properly, they will retain their medicinal potency for 3 to 5 years or even longer.

Making Herbal Preparations

Making your own herbal infusions, decoctions, and tinctures is easy. Herbal infusions and decoctions are basically teas prepared in a specific way to maximize the healing properties of the herb. They are similar to teas, in that the fresh or dried herb is steeped or simmered in hot water. Herbs are best prepared in glass, porcelain, earthenware, or enamel-coated steel pots. You can use stainless steel, but avoid aluminum or nonstick cookware.

I recommend drinking at least 3 cups of an herbal infusion or decoction daily during a cleansing program. Taking the herbs in liquid form helps to flush the kidneys and facilitates the removal of toxins from the body. I find it easiest to prepare a quart of herbal infusion or decoction fresh each morning, and then to drink it throughout the day, approximately 1 cup every 3 or 4 hours. Cleansing teas are most effective when taken warm or at room temperature, at least 15 minutes before a meal.

Herbal tinctures are made by steeping dried or fresh herbs in alcohol, vegetable glycerin, or vinegar for several weeks. Herbal tinctures are convenient to use and make it easy to take herbs that are not good tasting—gentian, for example. A typical dose of an herbal tincture is 30 drops 3 times daily. Dilute the tincture dosage in approximately 1/4 cup of hot water before taking.

How to Make an Herbal Infusion

If you've ever brewed a cup of herbal tea, you have made a simple herbal infusion. Infusions are used for the more delicate parts of the plant, such as the flowers, leaves, and seeds.

For a medicinal-strength infusion that retains all of the healing properties of the plant, use 1 to 2 teaspoons of dried herb per cup of water. If you are using fresh herbs, use 1 to 2 tablespoons. When using seeds, gently bruise them first to release the essential oils.

Pour boiling water over the herb and immediately cover the container to keep the volatile essential oils from escaping in the steam. Steep for 10 to 15 minutes and strain. For a stronger infusion, allow the herb to steep until the liquid cools to room temperature before straining. If you are making an infusion to use as a bath or steam inhalation, use 1 tablespoon of dried herb to each cup of water.

How to Make an Herbal Decoction

A decoction extracts the medicinal properties from the tougher parts of plants, typically the roots and barks. To make a decoction, place the herb in cold water in a covered pot. Use 1 to 2 teaspoons of dried herb to each cup of water. Slowly bring to a boil, lower the heat, and simmer for 15 to 20 minutes. Remove from the heat and strain. For a stronger decoction, allow the herb to steep until the liquid cools to room temperature before straining. As with an infusion, if you are making a decoction to use in a bath, increase the amount of herb to 1 tablespoon per cup of water.

How to Make Herbal Tinctures

To make an herbal tincture, you will need dried or fresh herbs and enough vodka to cover the herbs, plus 2 inches. Powder the dried herbs in a coffee grinder or blender. If using fresh herbs, chop them finely. Put the herbs into a glass jar with a tight-fitting lid and add the vodka. Cover, and keep in a warm, dark place for 2, or preferably 3 weeks. Shake the jar daily to thoroughly mix the herbs and vodka. After 3 weeks, strain the liquid through a colander or strainer lined with several layers of cheesecloth into a large bowl. Wring the herbs in the cheesecloth to extract any remaining liquid. Pour the tincture into dark glass bottles for storage.

Alcohol is the best liquid for extracting the medicinal properties of the herbs, but if you want to avoid alcohol, use vegetable glycerine or apple cider vinegar instead. To make a glycerine tincture using dried herbs, replace the vodka with a mixture of equal parts of vegetable glycerine and water. When making a tincture from fresh herbs, use a mixture of 3/4 vegetable glycerine and 1/4 water to adjust for the greater water content in the fresh plant.

To prepare a vinegar tincture, use undiluted natural apple cider vinegar and follow the basic directions for making a tincture. Because vinegar reacts with metal, place a piece of waxed paper over the jar before screwing on the lid.

HERBAL CLEANSING FORMULAS

Herbal Formulas to Enhance Digestion

Ginger Tea

According to Ayurvedic medicine, ginger tea is excellent for stimulating agni, *or digestive fire. At the same time, it reduces* ama, *or the accumulation of toxins in the digestive tract. Sip hot ginger tea after meals as a digestive aid. Ginger increases circulation and has antimicrobial properties, and is excellent for treating colds, flus and other respiratory problems, digestive ailments, and menstrual cramps. I drink ginger tea daily as a health tonic.*

3-4 teaspoons chopped fresh ginger root

1 teaspoon fennel seeds

1 teaspoon licorice root, if desired

Place herbs in a pot with 2 cups of water and simmer, covered, for 10 minutes. Strain. If you don't use licorice root, sweeten with honey if desired.

Herbal Bitters Tonic

Herbal bitters tonics are traditionally used for improving sluggish digestion and associated problems such as indigestion, flatulence, and constipation. Bitter herbs such as dandelion root and gentian stimulate the flow of digestive fluids, while ginger and fennel soothe the gastrointesti-

nal tract. Bitters tonics can be taken daily, and are especially helpful for improving the digestion of large meals or meals containing proteins and fats.

1/2 ounce dandelion root

1/4 ounce gentian root

1/4 ounce licorice root

1/4 ounce fennel seeds

1/4 ounce dried ginger root

1/4 ounce dried organic orange peel

1/4 ounce cardamom pods

vodka

Grind the herbs in a blender. Place in a glass jar and add enough vodka to cover the herbs, plus 2 inches. Close the jar tightly.

Place the jar in a warm, dark place, and give the jar a gentle shake every day or so to keep the herbs from settling. After 3 weeks, strain the liquid from the herbs through a colander or strainer lined with several layers of cheesecloth. Squeeze the herbs to strain out all of the liquid. Funnel your bitters tonic into a dark glass container, and store in a cool, dark place.

Take 1/2 to 1 teaspoonful of bitters tincture in 1/4 cup of warm water 15 to 30 minutes before eating.

After-Dinner Digestive Tea

Sipping a warm cup of herbal tea after meals is much healthier than drinking a cup of coffee. The following herbal tea is relaxing and promotes good digestion. Peppermint and anise have carminative properties (they help to relieve gas) and contain fragrant oils that stimulate digestion. Chamomile is a relaxant and contains mild bitter principles that enhance the flow of digestive fluids.

1 teaspoon peppermint

2 teaspoons chamomile

1 teaspoon anise seeds

Pour 2 cups of boiling water over the herbs. Cover, and let steep for 10 minutes. Strain, and drink while warm. Add honey and lemon if desired.

Herbal Formulas for the Liver

Sweet and Spicy Liver-Cleansing Tea

Dandelion, burdock, and Oregon grape root have bitter principles and are classic liver-cleansing herbs. Ginger and orange peel help to move stagnant energy in the liver. When simmered together, this makes a delicious tea that can be enjoyed daily during your cleansing program.

2 teaspoons dandelion root

2 teaspoons burdock root

2 teaspoons Oregon grape root

1 teaspoon ginger root

1 teaspoon fennel seeds

1 teaspoon organic orange peel

1 teaspoon licorice root

Place herbs and 1 quart of water in a covered pot. Bring to a boil over medium heat, lower the heat, and simmer for 15 minutes. Remove from heat and let steep an additional 15 minutes, or longer if desired. Strain and drink 3 to 4 cups throughout the day.

Purifying Aloe Drink

In Ayurvedic medicine, aloe is considered to be a rejuvenative for the liver. Western medicine has discovered that aloe has powerful healing properties for the entire gastrointestinal tract. Buy pure aloe vera juice that has no artificial additives or preservatives. "Green supplements" such as chlorella provide a boost of cleansing chlorophyll.

4 ounces aloe vera juice

4 ounces organic apple juice, if desired

1 teaspoon chlorella, spirulina, or powdered barley grass

pinch of powdered ginger

Mix all ingredients together and drink first thing in the morning.

Liver Tonic Capsules

Turmeric is a member of the ginger family and is a primary liver-cleansing herb in Ayurvedic medicine. It has powerful antioxidant prop-

erties and helps to protect the liver against toxins. It is also the main ingredient in curry powder. Turmeric seems to be absorbed best when taken with fats such as olive oil or ghee. Cultivate a taste for Indian cooking, or take these capsules with meals. Turmeric stains, so use care when putting these capsules together.

1/2 ounce powdered turmeric

1/2 ounce powdered ginger root

gelatin capsules, size OO

Mix the powdered herbs together in a deep, flat dish. Take the capsules apart, and fill the capsules by scooping the top and the bottom halves toward each other through the powdered herbs. Push the 2 halves together. Take 1 or 2 capsules twice daily with meals.

Liver-Strengthening Tincture

Dandelion, yellow dock, barberry, and Oregon grape root stimulate bile flow and are some of the best liver-cleansing herbs. Milk thistle seeds have the unique ability to stimulate liver regeneration. If you have a serious liver disease, avoid alcohol-based tinctures. Take milk thistle as a standardized extract or eat a couple of tablespoons of milk thistle seeds daily. They must be powdered to release their healing properties. Grind them in a coffee grinder and sprinkle onto hot cereal, salads, or soups.

1/2 ounce dandelion root

1/2 ounce milk thistle seeds

1/4 ounce barberry or Oregon grape root

1/4 ounce yellow dock root

1/4 ounce ginger root

1/4 ounce licorice root

vodka

Powder the herbs in a blender. Place in a clean glass jar and add enough vodka to cover herbs, plus 2 inches. Let steep in a warm, dark place and give the jar a gentle shake every day. After 3 weeks, strain the alcohol from the herbs through several layers of cheesecloth. Rebottle in a dark glass container, and store away from heat and light. Take 1 dropperful of tincture before meals 2 to 3 times daily in a small amount of warm water.

Herbal Formulas for the Large Intestine

Gentle Laxative Tea

Cascara sagrada is a gentle yet effective stimulant laxative. Licorice soothes the intestinal tract and has mild laxative properties, and ginger root helps to prevent any possible cramping.

1 teaspoon cascara sagrada bark

1/2 teaspoon licorice root

1/2 teaspoon ginger root

Place herbs in 1 cup of water. Bring to a boil, turn off the heat, and steep for 10 minutes. Strain, and drink before bed.

Laxative Tincture

This tincture is excellent for relieving occasional constipation. It's great to take along while traveling for sluggish bowels.

1/2 ounce cascara sagrada

1/2 ounce yellow dock root

1/2 ounce ginger root

1/2 ounce licorice root

vodka

Powder the herbs in a blender or coffee grinder. Place in a clean glass jar and add enough vodka to cover the herbs, plus 2 inches. Let steep in a warm, dark place and give the jar a gentle shake every day. After 3 weeks, strain the alcohol from the herbs through several layers of cheesecloth. Rebottle in a dark glass container, and store away from heat and light. Take 1 dropperful of tincture in a small amount of warm water before bed. Repeat the dosage in the morning if necessary.

Herbal Formulas for the Kidneys

Gentle Diuretic Tea

This tea is excellent for gently purifying the kidneys and for alleviating premenstrual water retention.

3 teaspoons dandelion leaf

3 teaspoons marshmallow root

1 teaspoon anise seeds, if desired for flavor

Pour 3 cups of boiling water over the herbs. Cover, and let steep until cool. Drink 3 cups throughout the day.

Antiseptic Diuretic Tincture

This tincture will help to relieve urinary tract infections. Take at the very first sign of an infection, usually burning upon urination and an increased need to urinate. In addition, drink at least 3 cups daily of Gentle Diuretic Tea, along with copious amounts of water to help flush out the bladder and urinary tract. Uva ursi, juniper berries, and yarrow all have potent antimicrobial properties.

1/4 ounce uva ursi

1/4 ounce juniper berries

1/4 ounce yarrow

1/4 ounce marshmallow root

vodka

Powder herbs in a blender. Place in a clean glass jar and add enough vodka to cover the herbs, plus 2 inches. Let steep in a warm, dark place and give the jar a gentle shake every day. After 3 weeks, strain the alcohol from the herbs through several layers of cheesecloth. Rebottle in a dark glass container, and store away from heat and light. Take 1 dropperful of tincture in a small amount of warm water 4 times daily at the first sign of an infection until the symptoms abate. If symptoms do not begin to subside within 24 hours, or if there is blood in the urine or fever, consult your health care practitioner.

Herbal Diaphoretic Formulas

Cooling Diaphoretic Tea

This tea is excellent for relieving a cold or flu. It is especially helpful for "hot" symptoms such as a fever, as it helps the body to naturally cool down by inducing perspiration, thus eliminating the virus.

2 teaspoons yarrow

2 teaspoons elder flower

2 teaspoons peppermint

1 teaspoon anise seeds, if desired for flavor

Pour 3 cups of boiling water over the herbs. Cover, and let steep for 10 minutes. Strain, and add honey and lemon if desired. Drink hot, 3 cups a day.

Warming Diaphoretic Tea

This is a wonderful tea for alleviating the chills and muscle soreness that often accompany a cold or flu. Ginger and cinnamon have warming properties and help to stimulate circulation.

2 tablespoons fresh ginger root, chopped

1 stick cinnamon, crushed

1 teaspoon fennel seeds, bruised

2 teaspoons licorice root if desired

Place the herbs into a pot along with 3 cups of water. Bring to a boil, and simmer, covered, for 10 minutes. Remove from heat and allow to steep for an additional 10 minutes. Strain, and if you don't use licorice, add honey if desired. Drink hot, up to 3 cups a day.

Lymphatic-Cleansing Formulas

Lymph-Purifying Tea

This gentle tea is an excellent tonic for the lymphatic system.

3 teaspoons cleavers

3 teaspoons red clover

1 teaspoon anise seeds, if desired for flavor

Pour 3 cups of boiling water over the herbs. Cover, and let steep until cool. Strain, and add honey and lemon if desired. Drink 3 cups daily.

Lymph-Purifying Tincture

This tincture is helpful to take during a cleansing program to purify the lymphatic fluid and to help to cleanse the lymph nodes. Echinacea and goldenseal have powerful antimicrobial properties.

1/2 ounce echinacea root

1/4 ounce goldenseal root

1/4 ounce prickly ash bark

vodka

Powder herbs in a blender. Place in a clean glass jar and add enough vodka to cover the herbs, plus 2 inches. Let steep in a warm, dark place and give the jar a gentle shake every day. After 3 weeks, strain the alco-

hol from the herbs through several layers of cheesecloth. Rebottle in a dark glass container, and store away from heat and light. Take 1 dropperful of tincture in a small amount of warm water 3 times daily for up to 2 weeks.

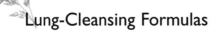

Lung-Cleansing Formulas

Lung-Cleansing Tea

This tea will help to relieve congestion related to colds, bronchitis, or allergies. It helps to soothe irritated bronchial passages and cleanses the lungs of excess mucus.

1 tablespoon mullein

1 tablespoon peppermint

1 tablespoon licorice root, if desired

Simmer licorice for 10 minutes in 3 cups of water. Add peppermint and mullein and steep for an additional 10 minutes. Strain, and if you don't use licorice, add honey if desired. Drink warm, 3 or more cups throughout the day.

Lung-Cleansing Tincture

This tincture is good for relieving chronic congestion and is helpful when taken with Lung-Cleansing Tea.

1/4 ounce thyme

1/4 ounce mullein

1/4 ounce fenugreek

1/4 ounce licorice root

1/4 ounce ginger

vodka

Powder herbs in a blender. Place in a clean glass jar and add enough vodka to cove the herbs, plus 2 inches. Let steep in a warm, dark place and give the jar a gentle shake every day. After 3 weeks, strain the alcohol from the herbs through several layers of cheesecloth. Rebottle in a dark glass container, and store away from heat and light. Take 1 dropperful before meals 2 to 3 times daily in a small amount of warm water.

Whole Body Cleansing Formulas

The following formulas are balanced to contain herbs which stimulate each organ of detoxification: the *liver, large intestine, kidneys, lymphatic system, lungs,* and *skin.* These are good detoxifying tea blends to use as a basis for your cleansing program.

Purifying Tea Blend #1

1 teaspoon burdock

1 teaspoon Oregon grape

1 teaspoon dandelion root

1 teaspoon licorice root

1 teaspoon nettle

1 teaspoon peppermint

1 teaspoon red clover

Combine burdock, Oregon grape, dandelion, and licorice with 3 cups of cold water. Bring to a boil in a covered pot over medium heat, reduce heat, and simmer for 15 minutes. Add nettle, peppermint, and red clover and steep for 10 minutes. Strain, and drink 3 cups throughout the day.

Purifying Tea Blend #2

1 teaspoon echinacea root

1 teaspoon dandelion root

1 teaspoon licorice root

1 teaspoon ginger root

1 teaspoon fenugreek seeds

1 teaspoon fennel seeds

1 teaspoon marshmallow root

Combine all ingredients in a covered pot and add 3 cups of cold water. Bring to a boil over medium heat, reduce heat, and simmer for 15 minutes. Remove from heat and let steep an additional 15 minutes. Strain, and drink 3 cups throughout the day.

chapter thirteen

Rejuvenate Your Body with a Natural Cleansing Diet

*B*ecause the cells of your body are created from the nutrients that you take in, the foods that you eat are an integral part of your detoxification program. From a purely physical aspect, you literally are what you eat. Your body is continually renewing itself, making new blood cells every day. In only four months, your entire bloodstream is replenished. The soft tissues of your body are made new approximately every three months, and your bone cells are replaced each year. Virtually your entire body is recreated every seven years. Each time you eat, you have an opportunity to improve your health and renew your body.

The Basics of a Cleansing Diet

A purifying diet provides your body with all of the nutrients it needs to function optimally, and also gives your body the opportunity to cleanse and rejuvenate. The healthiest diet is one that helps your body to detoxify on a daily basis. In addition to the foods you choose to eat, how and when you eat has a significant impact on your health. By choosing fresh, organic foods, not overeating, and including plenty of cleansing foods each day, you are giving your body the opportunity to keep up with daily maintenance. This allows for ongoing rejuvenation, which translates into increased energy, vitality, and health.

A purifying diet focuses on fresh, organic vegetables and fruits, complex carbohydrates in the form of whole grains and beans, easily digestible proteins, and healthy sources of essential fats. In addition to choosing health-supportive foods, avoiding foods which tend to create toxins is essential. Saturated and polyunsaturated fats, refined flour and sugar, processed foods, caffeine, alcohol, and excessive animal proteins place a burden on the liver and organs of elimination and cause impurities to build up in the body.

The healthier your daily diet, the less need you will have for drastic dietary measures. I frequently see people who pay virtually no attention to their diets for 51 weeks out of the year, and then decide to fast on nothing but water for a week. The results are almost always disastrous—they have unpleasant reactions such as headaches and fatigue and invariably break their fast with a radical binge on pizza and ice cream. Fasting can be a valuable tool for cleansing, but it is most effective when employed as part of an overall healthy approach to nourishing your body.

Purifying Diet Principles

Principle #1: Eat Organic Foods and Drink Pure Water

This is the first and most important principle. Pesticides, herbicides, and other poisonous agricultural chemicals in our food supply—and water—are a primary source of the toxins that we are exposed to. The liver and other organs of detoxification have difficulties breaking down and eliminating these substances; consequently, they end up stored in your body, where they damage cells, lay the groundwork for degenerative diseases, and cause premature aging.

Principle #2: Eat a Variety of Health Supportive Foods

Every person is unique, and each person's dietary needs will vary from day to day, depending on physical activity; climate, season, and weather; and emotional and physical demands. Vegetables, fruits, whole grains, legumes, nuts and seeds, fresh fish, organic poultry, some organic dairy products if desired (primarily yogurt and goat cheese), and healthy fats and oils (extra-virgin olive oil and small amounts of organic butter) form the basis of a health-enhancing diet. Eat a variety of foods to obtain a wide range of health-supportive nutrients, and let your choices come from your body's wisdom.

Principle #3: Eat an Abundance of Fresh Vegetables and Fruits

Fresh organic vegetables and fruits contain a variety of vitamins, minerals, and other protective substances that prevent the cell damage that leads to degenerative diseases and premature aging. In addition, fruits and vegetables are the most purifying foods for the body. Try to eat at least 5 servings of vegetables and 2 servings of fruits daily.

Principle #4: Eat Plenty of High-Fiber Foods

A fiber-rich diet speeds the removal of wastes from the body, and helps to naturally cleanse the intestinal tract. Soluble fiber (found in fruits, vegetables, legumes, and some grains and seeds) also helps to lower harmful cholesterol levels, and binds toxins in the intestinal tract to prevent their reabsorption into the bloodstream.

Principle #5: Avoid Congesting Foods

Certain foods are difficult for the body to digest and tend to create excess mucus and toxins, which interfere with healthy organ functioning. Saturated, polyunsaturated, and hydrogenated fats, most dairy products, baked flour products, refined and processed foods, sweets, and red meats are the primary offenders. Coffee and alcohol are are also dietary stressors, because they are drugs which must be detoxified by the liver. During a cleansing program, these foods are best avoided.

For optimal health, I recommend never eating polyunsaturated or hydrogenated fats, and limiting your intake of all other congesting or stressful foods. Don't become obsessed with eating a perfectly pure diet, but do pay attention to how you feel after eating certain foods. Good food is one of life's great pleasures, and I believe that eating should be an enjoyable experience. If you follow the basic principles of a cleansing diet on a daily basis, there's no reason to not enjoy a glass of wine or a special dessert on the weekend or at a party.

PRINCIPLES OF A PURIFYING DIET

Eat organic foods and drink pure water

Eat a variety of health-supportive foods

Eat an abundance of fresh fruits and vegetables

Eat plenty of high-fiber foods

Avoid congesting foods

Creating a Cleansing Diet

Understanding the principles of a health enhancing, cleansing diet will allow you to create the optimal diet for your needs. Follow the basic principles, and listen to your body. People vary in their dietary needs and preferences. For example, some people thrive on a primarily vegetarian diet, while others need animal protein daily to stay healthy. Be flexible and open to the messages that your body gives to you. The basic components of a detoxifying diet are fruits and vegetables, complex carbohydrates, lean proteins, and healthful oils. Each aspect is discussed in detail below.

Purify Your Body with Fresh Vegetables and Fruits

Fresh, organic vegetables and fruits are the primary components of a cleansing diet. They provide an abundance of vitamins and minerals as well as important phytonutrients that prevent cancer, heart disease, glaucoma, arthritis, and all other degenerative diseases. The soluble fiber in fresh fruits and vegetables cleanses the intestinal tract and arteries. Dark, leafy green vegetables such as watercress, romaine lettuce, and mustard greens are abundant in chlorophyll, which has natural detoxifying and cell-protective benefits. Deep orange and yellow vegetables and fruits and dark leafy greens contain powerful antioxidant vitamins that assist your body in neutralizing harmful free radicals and provide protection against cancer and other degenerative diseases. Sulfur-rich vegetables such as onions and garlic help to remove heavy metals from the body, and the cruciferous family, which includes broccoli, cabbage, and kale, blocks the formation of cancer-causing substances. In addition, fresh fruits and vegetables help to reduce excess acidity and bring the body into a healthy alkaline state.

Make it a goal to eat at least 5 servings of vegetables and 2 to 3 fruits daily. Increasing your intake of fresh produce is one of the most important dietary changes you can make. In general, consider 1/2 cup of cooked or raw vegetables, 1 cup of raw leafy greens, 1/2 cup or 1 piece of fresh fruit, or 1 cup of fresh vegetable or fruit juice as a serving. Vegetables and fruits with the deepest, richest colors are the best sources of protective antioxidants. For example, choose dark leafy greens over pale lettuces, and purple grapes over green grapes. Eat a variety of fruits and vegetables to obtain a wide range of protective nutrients, and eat them both both raw and cooked. While raw foods generally have the highest concentrations of antioxidants, some nutrients, like beta carotene, are most readily absorbed when vegetables are lightly cooked. Cook them so that they still have some crunch—and life force—left. Steaming, blanching, stir frying, and grilling are good cooking methods for preserving vital nutrients.

Although 5 servings of vegetables may sound like a lot, it's really not. For example, a mixed leafy green salad at lunch with marinated beans or a cup of bean and vegetable soup, a handful of raw baby carrots or a cup of carrot juice as a snack, and a baked potato and steamed broccoli at dinner provides 5 servings of vegetables. Don't limit yourself to 5 servings! Be creative and see how many vegetables you can eat in a day. I think of vegetables as the centerpiece of my diet, and try to make every lunch and dinner composed of at least 50 percent vegetables. You can't overdose on vegetables—every bite saturates your cells with health-protective nutrients.

In addition to eating at least 5 servings of vegetables daily, eat 2 to 3 servings of fresh fruits every day. As with vegetables, seek out the best and freshest organic fruits. Fruits provide natural, satisfying sweetness and are also the most purifying foods. They are quickly digested and have a natural laxative effect which cleanses the intestinal tract. Fresh fruit is an excellent way to begin the day and makes an ideal snack. Many people find that fruits are most easily digested when eaten in between meals. When eaten with meals, fruits—especially melons—tend to cause gas and bloating. Experiment and find out what works best for you.

Eat Complex Carbohydrates to Speed Cleansing

Whole grains and beans are rich sources of fiber, providing bulk that helps to naturally cleanse the intestinal tract. Fiber is an essential component of a cleansing and detoxification program. Pesticides, toxic metals, estrogen and other hormones, and a variety of other toxins are all swept out of the body by fiber. Through speeding up the movement of wastes through the intestines, fiber helps to detoxify the body. The longer that wastes remain in the body, the more opportunity toxins have for being reabsorbed into the bloodstream through the porous walls of the intestines. There are basically two types of fiber: *insoluble*, and *soluble*. Insoluble fiber is the indigestible part of plants, such as the outer husk of wheat. This type of fiber creates bulk and stimulates peristalsis, thereby expediting the removal of wastes from the body. Soluble fiber dissolves in water, and forms a gel-like substance in the intestinal tract. Barley, oats, and legumes are good examples of plants that are rich in soluble fiber. Soluble fiber absorbs toxic substances in the intestinal tract, helps to reduce cholesterol levels, and reduces bacterial toxins in the large intestine. Most plants contain a mixture of both types of fiber, but in varying amounts. For optimal health, eat a variety of whole grains and beans to obtain all of the cleansing protective benefits of fiber.

Complex carbohydrates are rich in B-complex vitamins and minerals. In addition, whole grains and beans are digested slowly, providing a steady flow of energy that keeps your blood sugar levels balanced throughout the day. Experiment with a variety of organic whole grains. Brown basmati rice is nutty and fragrant, quinoa cooks up fluffy and light, buckwheat is earthy and satisfying, and barley is a delicious, chewy addition to soups and stews. When choosing breads, look for whole grain breads that are made from freshly ground organic flours. While cleansing, you might want to pass up baked flour products such as breads in favor of whole grains. Flour products tend to be mucus producing, while whole grains are cleansing and provide bulk which helps to sweep out the intestinal tract. Avoid refined carbohydrates such as white bread and white rice—not only have they had all of their beneficial fiber stripped away, but also their vitamins and minerals. Eating refined pasta or white rice on an occasional basis will do you no harm, but make a conscious effort to eat whole grains every day to supply your body with their detoxifying and health-enhancing benefits. Try to eat at least 2 servings of complex carbohydrates daily, figuring approximately 1/2 cup of cooked grains or beans as one serving.

Complex carbohydrates, especially beans, also contain other health-protective substances called *protease inhibitors*, natural enzymes that inhibit carcinogens in the intestinal tract. Many people have difficulty digesting beans because of complex sugars that require specific digestive enzymes. Eating beans frequently will help you to digest them more easily. Begin with small amounts to give your body an opportunity to adjust and be sure to cook them properly. You can eliminate most of the problematic sugars in beans with the following method: Soak beans for at least 4 hours (preferably overnight) and pour off the soaking water. Add fresh water, bring to a boil, and simmer until tender.

Rejuvenate Your Body with Protein

Proteins provide your body with the building blocks it needs for restoration and rejuvenation. Too much protein stresses your body, causing a build-up of uric acid in the bloodstream that the kidneys have to eliminate. But your body needs protein to keep your muscles strong, your skin and hair healthy, and for the repair of tissues and organs. For most people, 6- to 8-ounces of protein daily is sufficient.

Some proteins are better for the body than others. Fish, poultry, and tofu are more easily digested than red meats. Tofu and fish also have other health benefits that make them a valuable addition to the diet. Fish, especially fatty fish such as salmon, tuna, sardines, mackerel, and herring, are rich in omega-3 fatty acids, which play a variety of protective roles in the body. Omega-3 oils keep the arteries clean and flexible and thin the blood, preventing the formation of dangerous blood clots. They also lower triglycerides and raise levels of beneficial HDL cholesterol and help to reduce blood pressure. Omega-3 oils offer protection against degenerative diseases such as arthritis, cancer, diabetes, and skin diseases such as eczema and pso-riasis. Seafood is also rich in selenium and coenzyme Q-10, 2 potent antioxidants that protect cells from degenerative changes. To reap the benefits of the omega-3 oils found in fish, eat several 4-ounce servings of fatty fish per week.

Soybeans are not only an excellent source of complete veg-etable protein, but are loaded with protective antioxidants. Soybeans help to protect cells from free radical damage and contain powerful natural chemicals that help to prevent cancer. One of the most potent antioxidants in soybeans is *genistein*, which is protective against cancer, atherosclerosis, heart attacks, and strokes. Soybeans help to cleanse the arteries by increasing levels of good HDL choles-terol and blocking the oxidation of LDL cholesterol, the harmful cholesterol which damages arteries. They also help to regulate blood sugar levels. Soybeans are available in a variety of forms, including tofu, tempeh, soy milk, and soy protein. To obtain the full health-protective benefits of soy, eat 3 to 4 ounces of tofu or tempeh daily, or 1 cup of soy milk. Use soy milk as you would regular milk—on morning cereal, in blender drinks, or in cooking and baking.

While dairy products are good sources of protein as well as cal-cium, they tend to be difficult for many people to digest and are common dietary allergen. In addition, dairy products create conges-tion and excess mucus. The least stressful dairy foods are goat milk and goat cheeses, and yogurt, which is beneficial because it helps to replenish healthy intestinal flora.

Protect Your Health with Essential Fatty Acids

Although the trend in recent years has been toward low-fat diets, the truth is that fats are essential for health. Eating the wrong types of fat damages cells, causes cancer and heart disease, and speeds up the aging process. But eating healthy fats provides pro-tection against cancer, heart disease, and other degenerative diseases, and helps to keep you young.

Unhealthy fats include *polyunsaturated oils, saturated fats,* and *hydrogenated oils.* Polyunsaturated oils such as safflower, corn, sesame, soybean, and sunflower oils are extremely detrimental to your health. They quickly oxidize when exposed to oxygen and cre-ate free radicals, mutant molecules that destroy healthy cells.

Polyunsaturated oils become even more toxic when they undergo the process of hydrogenation to become margarine or shortening. Trans-fatty acids are created during this process, an unnatural and dangerous fat that impairs healthy cell function, clogs arteries, lowers beneficial HDL cholesterol, depresses the immune system, and stimulates the growth of cancer. Don't eat these fats or any processed or packaged foods made with them. Not only are they sources of harmful free radicals, but once inside the body, they continue to oxidize and create more free radicals. In addition to eliminating polyusaturated oils and hydrogenated fats, also cut down on saturated fats, found primarily in red meat, whole milk dairy products, poultry skin, and palm and coconut oil. These fats cause an increase in unhealthy blood cholesterol, clog the arteries, and greatly increase the risk of cardiovascular disease.

The healthiest form of fat is extra-virgin olive oil. Olive oil is a *monounsaturated oil*, and slow to oxidize. In addition, it offers a variety of health-protective benefits. Olive oil reduces harmful LDL cholesterol levels and at the same time raises levels of protective HDL cholesterol. It helps to cleanse the blood of excess cholesterol, and contains natural substances that prevent the formation of dangerous blood clots. Olive oil also makes cell membranes more resistant to the destructive effects of free radicals, and helps to prevent heart disease and cancer. While peanut and canola oils are also monounsaturated oils, peanut oil is often contaminated with pesticide residues and contains naturally occuring toxins. Canola oil, made from rapeseed, is also likely to be contaminated with pesticides and is extracted with toxic solvents. Organic expeller-pressed canola oil is available at natural foods stores, and some people like using it because it is virtually flavorless. However, it does not have the health-protective benefits of olive oil. The only fats in my kitchen are extra-virgin olive oil, organic ghee, and organic butter. I love the flavor of good olive oil, and use it for salads and sautéing. For occasional baking, I use organic butter or ghee, which is clarified butter. According to Ayurvedic medicine, ghee has health-protective properties and helps the body to eliminate toxins that are stored in the fatty tissues.

A good general guideline is to keep your total level of dietary fat to approximately 20 percent of your daily caloric intake. Make sure that you're getting plenty of the beneficial omega-3 fatty acids, found in oily fish, such as salmon, tuna, and sardines, and in some vegetable foods, primarily flaxseeds, walnuts, and soybeans. Vegetable sources of omega-3 fatty acids are less potent than fish oils, but are a good alternative for vegetarians. In addition, eat foods rich in *glutathione*, primarily found in fresh fruits and vegetables, a powerful antioxidant which helps to protect the body from rancid fats.

Nineteen Cleansing Foods from the Garden

Science is finally beginning to acknowledge that food truly is our best medicine. Fresh fruits and vegetables contain an abundance of vitamins and minerals, as well as a variety of beneficial natural substances that protect the cells from changes that lead to cancer, heart disease, and other degenerative diseases. Fruits and vegetables are also nature's most potent cleansing foods. The high soluble fiber content of fresh produce helps to cleanse the intestinal tract and also helps to reduce levels of harmful LDL cholesterol in the bloodstream. Because of their rich mineral content, fruits and vegetables help to restore the blood to a healthy alkaline balance. Many fruits and vegetables have gentle diuretic or laxative properties, as well. Following are some examples of fruits and vegetables with powerful cleansing and healing properties.

Apples

The old saying "An apple a day keeps the doctor away" is folk wisdom that has a strong scientific basis. Apples are rich in *pectin*, a water-soluble fiber that sweeps through the large intestine and binds with cholesterol to help to cleanse the blood of harmful LDL cholesterol. Eating just 2 apples a day is sufficient to significantly lower cholesterol levels. In addition, apples contain caffeic acid, a potent anticancer agent. To obtain the full health-protective benefits of apples, be sure to eat the whole apple, including the skin. Try *Carrot-Apple Salad* (p. 160) and *Apples Poached with Cinnamon and Vanilla* (p. 182).

Asparagus

Fresh asparagus is a classic "spring tonic" vegetable. As one of the first vegetables to appear in the spring, it helps to cleanse the body of toxins that have accumulated over the winter. Asparagus contains the amino acid *asparagine*, which has a diuretic effect and is an excellent kidney-purifying tonic. In addition, asparagus is rich in vitamin C, vitamin A, folic acid, potassium, and rutin, a bioflavonoid which helps to strengthen the capillaries. Try *Asparagus with Roasted Red Peppers* (p. 161) and *Asparagus with Lemon.*

Beets

Beets are a rich storehouse of minerals, including iron, potassium, copper, zinc, calcium, and magnesium. Because they are a good source of soluble fiber, they help to cleanse the large intestine and have a natural laxative effect. Raw beets are delicious when finely grated with an equal part of carrots and dressed with olive oil and fresh orange juice. Their high natural iron content makes them a good blood builder. Try *Citrus Beet Salad* (p. 159).

Broccoli

Broccoli, one of the best loved cruciferous vegetables, is a rich source of beta-carotene and other carotenoids, along with a variety of other powerful antioxidants that neutralize free radicals. Eating broccoli regularly—several times a week—has been shown to lower the risk of a variety of cancers, including cancer of the colon, lung, prostate, and stomach. Broccoli is also a good source of B-complex vitamins, sulfur, iron, and chlorophyll, and has more vitamin C than citrus fruits. Try quick-boiling broccoli for the best flavor and retention of nutrients. Bring a pot of water to a boil—just enough to barely cover the broccoli—and add fresh broccoli, cover, and cook at a rapid boil until crisply tender. Try *Broccoli and White Bean Salad* (p. 162) and *Sauteed Tempeh with Broccoli* (p. 170).

Burdock

Burdock root is a classic liver tonic herb that finds its way into almost all of my purifying liver tea and tincture blends. In addition, the fresh root is one of my favorite vegetables. Rich in minerals, B-complex vitamins, and vitamins C and E, burdock helps to cleanse the blood through its action on the liver, and its gentle diuretic properties promote the elimination of toxins through increased kidney function. Oriental groceries carry fresh burdock root, as do many natural foods stores, or you can dig your own from the wild with the help of a good plant identification book (see Resources p. 284). The earthy, rich flavor of burdock is a delicious addition to soups and vegetable stews. Try *Autumn Tonic Soup* (p. 167).

Cabbage

Cabbage, another member of the cruciferous vegetable family, also has powerful cancer-preventive properties. Cabbage contains a variety of potent anticancer agents such as *indoles, chlorophyll,* and *flavonoids* that block the development of cancerous cells. Eating raw or cooked cabbage only once a week has been shown to reduce the risk of colon cancer by more than sixty percent. Enjoy cabbage in all its forms, including purple, bok choy, and Chinese (or Napa) cabbage. Naturally fermented and unpasteurized sauerkraut is an excellent source of beneficial bacteria and is helpful for improving the health of intestinal flora. Try *Cabbage Apple Walnut Salad* (p. 159) and *Cabbage Tofu Rolls* (p. 169).

Carrots

Carrots are one of the best sources of beta-carotene, with approximately 5,000 units of this health-protective nutrient in one carrot and 25,000 units of beta-carotene—an entire day's health protective allowance—in one cup of fresh carrot juice. Beta-carotene promotes healthy liver function, and has powerful antioxidant properties, which protects cells from the damaging changes that are the primary cause of degenerative diseases. Carrots are also rich in pectin, which helps to alleviate constipation, cleanse the colon, and lower blood cholesterol levels. Try *Carrot Soup with Dill* (p. 166), and *Carrot-Apple Salad* (p. 160).

Cherries

Cherries are often recommended for alleviating the painful symptoms of arthritis, gout, and rheumatism. They relieve rheumatic complaints by neutralizing excess acids in the body and alkalizing the blood. The gentle laxative effect of cherries makes them excellent for cleansing the intestinal tract. Cherries are good sources of vitamin A and C, and are rich in minerals, which makes them helpful for building the blood. They also are a good source of *ellagic acid* which has cancer-preventive properties.

Garlic

Garlic has powerful antimicrobial properties and helps to cleanse the body of a variety of unhealthy microorganisms, including bacteria, fungi, viruses, and parasites. To obtain the antimicrobial benefits, garlic must be eaten raw, either chopped or crushed. Add raw garlic to salad dressings or to soups or pasta dishes just before serving. Garlic also enhances the functioning of the immune system, and helps to cleanse the blood of harmful LDL cholesterol, while increasing levels of beneficial HDL cholesterol. In addition, garlic thins the blood and helps to prevent blood clots. To enjoy all of the health-protective benefits of this wonderful herb, eat 2 or 3 cloves daily, both raw and cooked. If you're concerned about garlic breath, chew on a sprig of parsley or a few fennel seeds. Try *Garlic Mashed Potatoes* (p. 175).

Grapes

The diuretic and intestinal-cleansing properties of grapes make them an ideal snack as part of a detoxifying program. Grapes contain *caffeic acid*, a natural compound which has potent anticancer benefits, and a wide variety of other antioxidants. Because these protective nutrients are concentrated in grape skins, red and purple grapes are richer in antioxidants than green grapes. Grapes are good sources of potassium and vitamin C, and the darker varieties in particular are rich in iron and help to build healthy blood. In addition, grape juice is beneficial for the cardiovascular system, helping to lower blood levels of harmful LDL cholesterol and to increase beneficial levels of HDL cholesterol.

Grapefruit

Grapefruit are an excellent source of pectin, the soluble fiber that helps to sweep out the intestines and lower blood cholesterol levels. In addition to cleansing the blood of harmful excess cholesterol, fresh grapefruit contain a natural chemical that helps to dissolve cholesterol plaques in arteries. Like all citrus fruits, grapefruit are rich in vitamin C, which has potent antioxidant properties and is protective against cancer. The white inner rind is high in bioflavonoids, which strengthens the capillaries. The slightly sour taste of grapefruit stimulates liver function and purifies the digestive tract. To obtain the full benefits of grapefruit, eat whole grapefruit, including the pulp and some of the white inner rind. Grapefruit are also a good source of *glutathione*, a powerful antioxidant that protects the cells from damage by oxidized fats. Try *Avocado Grapefruit Salad* (p. 162).

Kale

Dark, leafy green kale has the highest content of carotenoids of all of the leafy green vegetables. Carotenoids, including beta carotene, are powerful antioxidants, and help to protect the body against cancer and other degenerative diseases. Chlorophyll, vitamin C, calcium, magnesium, folic acid, and iron are found in abundance in kale. The calcium in kale is easily absorbed, which makes it valuable for those who choose to avoid dairy products or who must because of lactose intolerance. My favorite way of preparing kale is to lightly sauté the chopped leaves in olive oil with fresh garlic or ginger. Try *Kale with Currants and Pumpkin Seeds* (p. 174).

Lemon

Lemons are excellent for cleansing the digestive tract and for helping to alkalize the blood. In Chinese medicine, the sour taste of lemon taken in moderation is believed to be beneficial for the liver. Lemons, like other citrus fruits, are rich in vitamin C, which acts as an antioxidant to protect body cells. Lemon and other citrus fruit rinds also contain a substance called *limonene* which has potent anti-cancer properties. To take advantage of the protective properties of limonene, add the zest of fresh organic lemon or oranges to salad dressings, soups, or sauces and simmer slices of lemon or orange peel in herbal tea blends. Try starting the day with a glass of filtered water with a squeeze of fresh lemon juice. Lemon stimulates intestinal function and the astringent properties help to cleanse the body of excess mucus.

Onion

The humble onion has a variety of health-protective and cleansing benefits. The pungent flavor of onions helps to improve circulation and reduce excess mucus in the respiratory tract and throughout the body. They are rich in sulfur, which promotes detoxification from heavy metals and parasites. Natural compounds in onions help to regulate blood pressure and eliminate damaging LDL cholesterol while increasing levels of beneficial HDL cholesterol. For the most powerful benefits, eat onions both raw and cooked. Red and yellow onions contain *quercetin*, a potent antioxidant that neutralizes carcinogens and has antimicrobial and anti-inflammatory properties. Try *Onion and Red Pepper Confit* (p. 178).

Parsley

Fresh parsley deserves more attention than just as an occasional garnish to a meal. Parsley contains an abundance of vitamin A, vitamin C, iron, calcium, and magnesium and is a rich source of cleansing chlorophyll. It stimulates increased urination and helps to purify the urinary tract. Add liberal amounts of fresh minced parsley to salads, soups, and pasta dishes. I often combine fresh parsley with carrots and apples for a delicious and refreshing juice tonic. Try *Hummus with Parsley* (p. 181).

Pineapple

Fresh pineapple contains *bromelain*, a digestive enzyme that not only aids digestion, but also has potent anti-inflammatory properties. Although many people find it easiest to digest fruits if they are eaten either 30 minutes before or 2 hours after meals, the digestive-enhancing properties of pineapple make it beneficial when eaten as an appetizer or dessert. Eating fresh pineapple between meals helps to cleanse the body of accumulations of mucus and other metabolic wastes. Avoid underripe acidic pineapple, and choose those which are ripe, sweet, and juicy.

Spinach

Spinach is rich in beta-carotene and other carotenoids, which have potent antioxidant properties and help to protect the body against degenerative cell changes. A potent natural chemical in spinach is *lutein*, which is as powerful an antioxidant as beta carotene. In addition, the high concentration of chlorophyll in spinach blocks the formation of cancer-causing substances in the gastrointestinal tract. Spinach is a good blood builder because of its abundant iron content. To preserve vitamins and help neutralize oxalic acid, which interferes with calcium absorption, cook spinach quickly in a small amount of boiling water. Try *Spinach with Sesame Seeds* (p. 175).

Watercress

Slightly spicy watercress is an exceptionally rich source of calcium, iron, and carotenoids. The high chlorophyll content of watercress makes it an excellent blood purifier, and the slightly bitter taste is helpful for stimulating liver and gall bladder function. Add chopped fresh watercress to soups at the last minute, or toss a handful into a leafy green salad for a refreshing pungent flavor. Watercress also has diuretic properties and can be made into a tea by steeping 1 tablespoon of chopped fresh herb in 1 cup of boiling water for 10 minutes. Try watercress with *Orange Vinaigrette* (p. 163).

Watermelon

Sweet, juicy watermelon is a delicious summer treat that cleanses and cools the body. Watermelon has excellent diuretic properties and helps to purify the kidneys. In addition, watermelon is rich in beta-carotene, vitamin C, potassium, and magnesium. Watermelon is easily digested, but only if eaten alone. When combined with other foods, melons tend to cause bloating and intestinal gas. Watermelon is one of the few foods (tomatoes are another) that contain *lycopene*, a potent antioxidant that may be even more powerful than beta carotene.

Special Detoxifying Foods

The following foods have special detoxifying benefits. Emphasize them during a cleansing program, and include them in your diet regularly to maintain optimal health.

Calcium-Rich Foods

Foods high in calcium help the body to detoxify in a number of ways. They assist in eliminating toxic heavy metals, and block the absorption of saturated fats in the gastrointestinal tract which helps to lower levels of harmful LDL cholesterol. Calcium also helps to protect against the formation of cancerous cells. Other health benefits of calcium include maintaining bone and cardiovascular health, and relieving symptoms of anxiety and stress. Try to get between 1,000 and 2,000 milligrams of calcium daily. Although dairy products are rich in calcium, many people have difficulties digesting them, and dairy foods tend to be congesting. Fortunately, calcium is found in a wide variety of foods. Eat plenty of high-calcium foods daily, and take a calcium supplement if necessary. Avoid calcium supplements made from bone meal or dolomite because they may be contaminated with lead. Choose supplements made from calcium citrate or calcium carbonate, and take them with meals for optimum absorption. For calcium-rich recipes, try *Sauteed Greens with Garlic* (p. 174), *Tahini Orange Sauce* (p. 181), and *Marinated Grilled Tofu* (p. 172).

CALCIUM-RICH FOODS

Almonds

Broccoli

Collards

Kale

Legumes

Oranges

Sesame seeds

Tofu

Sardines

Vitamin C-Rich Foods

Vitamin C is abundant in a wide variety of fruits and vegetables, but many people don't even get the 60 milligrams a day that is needed for the body just to perform its basic functions. Vitamin C acts in a number of ways to cleanse and protect the body. It helps to prevent cancer by shielding cells from damaging free radicals, it enhances immune function, and blocks the formation of carcinogens in the intestinal tract by stimulating the production of glutathione, a potent antioxidant. Vitamin C also protects the cardiovascular system by increasing beneficial HDL cholesterol, cleansing the arteries, strengthening blood vessels, and preventing blood clots.

In addition to eating a variety of vegetables and fruits every day, take an additional 1,000 milligrams of vitamin C as a daily supplement. Divide into 2 or 3 doses to keep the cells well supplied. For vitamin C-rich recipes, try *Arugula Orange Salad* (p. 160), *Fresh Tomato, Corn, and Black Bean Salad* (p. 162), *Salsa Fresca* (p. 179), and *Peaches in Strawberry Sauce* (p. 182).

VITAMIN C-RICH FRUITS AND VEGETABLES

Broccoli

Cantaloupe

Cauliflower

Grapefruit

Kiwi

Lemons

Oranges

Papaya

Peaches

Red bell peppers

Strawberries

Tomatoes

Carotene-Rich Foods

Carotenoids, including beta carotene, have powerful antioxidant properties that protect the cells against degenerative changes. They inhibit the formation of cancerous cells, prevent the build-up of plaque in arteries, and stimulate immune function. Beta carotene and other carotenoids are abundant in fresh fruits and vegetables.

For health-protective benefits, try to get 25,000 units of beta carotene daily. A cup of carrot juice contains almost that amount, and if you eat 5 servings of fresh vegetables and a couple of servings of fresh fruits daily, you should be able to easily meet your daily requirement. For carotene-rich recipes, try *Red Peppers Stuffed with Rice, Corn, and Basil* (p. 176), *Mango Salsa* (p. 179), *Spinach with Sesame Seeds* (p. 175), and *Sweet Winter Squash Soup* (p. 168).

CAROTENE-RICH FRUITS AND VEGETABLES

Apricots

Broccoli

Cantaloupe

Carrots

Collard greens

Dandelion greens

Kale

Mango

Peaches

Red bell peppers

Romaine lettuce

Spinach

Sweet potatoes

Tomatoes

Watermelon

Winter squash

Glutathione-Rich Foods

Glutathione is an amino acid found in a variety of foods, and is also produced by every cell in the body. It is a potent antioxidant, and plays a critical role in detoxification. Glutathione helps to neutralize and break down free radicals so that they can be eliminated by the body. It destroys oxidized fats in the gastrointestinal tract, a primary cause of free radicals, and is protective against a wide variety of degenerative diseases, including cancer, arthritis, diabetes, and heart disease. Glutathione also helps to strengthen and regenerate immune cells. For glutathione-rich recipes, try *Asparagus with Lemon* (p. 178), *Avocado Grapefruit Salad, Broccoli and White Bean Salad* (p. 162), and *Garlic Mashed Potatoes* (p. 175).

GLUTATHIONE-RICH FOODS

Asparagus

Avocado

Broccoli

Cauliflower

Grapefruit

Onions

Oranges

Potatoes

Strawberries

Tomatoes

Watermelon

Guidelines for a Health Enhancing Diet

- 5 or more servings of fresh vegetables
  (emphasize dark leafy green and deep orange vegetables and cruciferous vegetables such as broccoli and cabbage)
- 2 or more servings of fresh fruits
- 2 or more servings of complex carbohydrates
  (emphasize soluble-fiber-rich whole grains and legumes)
- 2 3-to 4-ounce servings of lean protein
  (eat fish often for omega-3 oils, and tofu and tempeh for their potent cancer-preventive properties)
- 2 tablespoons olive oil

- several servings per week of omega-3 oils
  (found in fatty fish, flax seeds, walnuts)
- emphasize special cleansing foods: foods rich in calcium, vitamin C, carotenes, and glutathione

Fasting

A 1 to 3 day juice fast can be helpful for alkalizing body tissues and giving the digestive system a rest. By flushing your cells with fresh fruits and vegetables in juice form, you saturate your body with antioxidants and other cleansing and protective nutrients.

In general, eating a health-enhancing diet with occasional short fasts of 1 to 3 days is a safe and effective path to detoxification. Many natural health practitioners recommend cultivating the practice of fasting 1 day each week as a way of purifying and healing the body. Some people enjoy fasting 3 days each month, and others fast from 1 to 3 days in the early spring and again in the early fall at the time when the seasons are changing and the body naturally wants to detoxify. In Ayurvedic medicine and other traditional forms of healing, the most auspicious times for cleansing are around the times of the Spring and Autumn equinoxes. If you listen to your body, it will let you know when you need to cleanse. While cleansing has powerful health benefits, just like anything else, it can be taken to an extreme. Do not attempt a fast of longer than 3 days without the consent of your health practitioner.

Do not fast if you are pregnant or nursing, or if you have any serious health condition without first consulting your health practitioner.

Brief juice fasts give the digestive organs a rest and allow the body to focus its energy on cleansing and rejuvenation. During a fast, the body steps up its process of detoxification. While some health practitioners advocate a water fast, I find that most people fare better when they fast on juices. Juices contain natural sugars which make fasting easier and provide energy, and they also supply an abundance of vitamins, minerals, and phytonutrients that enhance the cleansing process. They are also excellent sources of natural enzymes which aid in digestion and help to cleanse the blood, tissues, and organs of excess acids, fats, and metabolic wastes.

Juice fasting is most appropriate in the spring and summer when the weather is warm and plenty of fresh organic produce is available. Drink 6 or more 8-ounce glasses of freshly squeezed vegetable and fruit juices throughout the day, diluted with 1/3 water. To obtain a full range of healing nutrients, consume a variety of fresh juices. In addition, to promote thorough cleansing of your cells, drink at least 1 quart of purified water or a cleansing herbal tea each day that you are fasting.

During the late fall and winter months, it's helpful to give your body an occasional rest from the normal processes of digestion, but fast on warm vegetable broths, light vegetable soups, and steamed vegetables instead of juices. Unless you live in a very warm climate, a juice fast tends to be debilitating instead of cleansing during the cooler months. A bit of miso added to soups helps to replenish healthy intestinal flora, and ginger and garlic add warming cleansing benefits. Try *Miso Shiitake Soup* (p. 165) or *Autumn Tonic Soup* (p. 167). Consume 3 to 4 bowls of soup throughout the day during a cleanse, along with a variety of steamed vegetables. Drink an additional quart of warm herbal tea and hot water with lemon daily while you are fasting.

Many people find that they enjoy fasting on a weekend, when they can devote their full attention to cleansing and rejuvenating activities. While fasting, you should plan to keep your life as simple as possible. Choose a time when you have fewer responsibilities and can relax. Gentle walks in the fresh air and stretching exercises will stimulate cleansing, but avoid strenuous exercise. Spend time outdoors, and enjoy a moderate amount of early morning or late afternoon sunlight. A sauna or other detoxifying bath will help to purify your body. Be sure to drink plenty of fluids as well as juices, and get plenty of rest. You may find that you require less sleep than normal during a fast, but still take time to slow down and relax, and your body will reward you with increased vitality.

Most people find that they feel immediately lighter and clearer during a fast. You may experience minor "cleansing reactions" such as fatigue or a slight headache, although these symptoms are less likely to occur with a juice fast than with a water fast. Be sure to take extra fiber such as psyllium husks during a fast, and to drink 2 to 3 quarts of liquids each day. If desired, you can also take an herbal laxative each evening before bed to speed the elimination of toxins. Discontinue any supplements while fasting except for vitamin C, which helps the body to detoxify.

Break a fast gently. The morning after a fast, eat a breakfast of fruit, and make lunch an easily digestible meal of a variety of vegetables and a light protein such as tofu or fish.

Sample Fasting Program

- The night before beginning your fast, eat a simple meal with plenty of fresh vegetables and easily digested protein such as tofu or fish. Drink a cup of Gentle Laxative Tea (p. 130) before going to sleep.

- Upon rising, drink a glass of pure water with a squeeze of fresh lemon or lime juice. Follow 15 minutes later with a glass of Intestinal Cleansing Beverage (p. 81).

- One-half hour later, drink a glass of fresh fruit or vegetable juice. Every two to three hours, drink a glass of fresh fruit or vegetable juice, for a total of 6 8-ounce glasses of juice throughout the day. In between, sip on Herbal Purifying Tea (p. 134) or purified water.

- Take a gentle walk in nature, do some stretching or yoga, and spend time resting and relaxing. Get a bit of sunshine and a lot of fresh air to nourish your body and your spirit.

- Enjoy a massage and a sauna or purifying bath (see Chapter 15) to support your body's detoxification.

- Go to bed early to allow your body to continue its cleansing work. Continue your fast for up to 3 days if desired.

- Break your fast with a breakfast of Gingered Fruit Compote (p. 182) or fresh fruit, and make lunch a simple and healthful combination of a variety of vegetables and easily digested proteins and carbohydrates.

Purifying Juices

Apple juice: Rich in vitamins and minerals, apple juice also contains large amounts of pectin which helps to sweep toxins from the intestinal tract. Apples combine well with other juices.

Beets: The high mineral content of beets helps to cleanse and build the blood. Beet juice is potent and is best mixed with other juices such as carrot or apple. Combine one or two ounces of beet juice with six ounces of other juice.

Cabbage: Cabbage juice is rich in vitamin C and purifying sulfur. It also contains vitamin U, which is recommended as a treatment for stomach ulcers. To prevent intestinal gas, dilute cabbage juice with other vegetable juices.

Carrot: Carrot juice is an excellent source of health-protective beta carotene, and is also high in calcium and other minerals. Carrot juice is rich in pectin and stimulates liver and intestinal cleansing. Add greens such as parsley or kale or a squeeze of lemon to balance the intense sweetness of carrots.

Celery: The high mineral content of celery helps to calm the nervous system. Celery has a slightly salty taste that is good mixed in small amounts with sweet vegetables like carrots and beets.

Cherry: Cherries are a good source of vitamins A and C, and help to alkalize the blood. Cherry juice reduces excess acidity and is recommended for gout or arthritis. Because it is extremely sweet, cherry juice is best mixed with other fruit juices or diluted with water.

Cranberry: Cranberry juice has natural diuretic properties and helps to cleanse the urinary tract. It is useful for relieving urinary tract infections. Cranberry juice is very tart and should be mixed with sweet fruit juices.

Cucumber: Cucumber has cooling, natural diuretic properties and helps to cleanse the urinary tract. Cucumber juice is also rich in potassium and other minerals.

Dandelion greens: Dandelion greens are a classic spring tonic and are rich in beta carotene and minerals. The bitter flavor stimulates bile flow and helps to cleanse the liver. If you pick your own, choose tender young leaves that appear in the early spring. Add a small amount of dandelion juice to vegetable juice combinations.

Grapefruit: Pink and red grapefruit are the sweetest choices and are less acidic than white grapefruit. Grapefruit juice is rich in vitamin C and bioflavonoids. Leave some of the white rind on the fruit when juicing to obtain all the protective nutrients.

Kale: Dark leafy green kale is rich in calcium, iron, and cleansing chlorophyll as well as beta carotene. Add small amounts to sweet vegetable juices.

Lemon: Lemons are an excellent source of vitamin C and bioflavonoids. The sour taste of lemon helps to purify the liver, and it encourages intestinal cleansing by stimulating peristalsis. Add small amounts to any fruit or vegetable juice.

Parsley: Parsley is rich in beta carotene, vitamin C, chlorophyll, and minerals. It is an excellent blood cleanser and also has diuretic properties. Parsley juice is potent and is best used in small amounts mixed with other juices.

Watermelon: Watermelon, seeds included, is a wonderful diuretic. It cleanses the bladder and kidneys while eliminating excess fluids from the body. Watermelon is also a good source of beta carotene. To avoid gastric discomfort, do not mix with other juices.

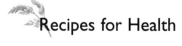

Recipes for Health

Salads

Cabbage Apple Walnut Salad

Cabbage contains an abundance of cancer-preventive phytonutrients. This salad is best if allowed to stand for 2 to 3 hours before serving to give the cabbage time to soften. Serves 4.

4 cups finely shredded green cabbage

2 scallions, finely minced

1 apple, diced

1/4 cup walnuts, chopped coarsely

2 tablespoons extra virgin olive oil

2 tablespoons freshly squeezed lemon juice

sea salt to taste

1. Combine cabbage with scallions, olive oil, lemon juice, and sea salt. Mix well and allow to stand for 2 to 3 hours before serving.

2. Add diced apple and walnuts just before serving, and adjust seasonings.

Citrus Beet Salad

Lemon and orange add a refreshing tanginess and bring out the natural sweetness of beets. Beets are rich in cleansing fiber and also help to build healthy red blood cells. Serves 4.

1 pound beets

juice of 1 large orange

1 tablespoon lemon juice

1 teaspoon maple syrup

2 tablespoons extra virgin olive oil

1 tablespoon grated orange peel

1 tablespoon finely chopped fresh mint

sea salt to taste

1. Simmer beets in a large pot of water for approximately 30 minutes, or until they can be pierced with a knife. Remove from water and cool. 2. Peel beets and slice into 1/2-inch slices. Combine orange juice, lemon juice, maple syrup, olive oil, grated orange peel, mint, and sea salt. Pour over beets and marinate for 1 hour before serving. Adjust seasonings and serve.

Arugula Orange Salad

Arugula is a delicious salad green with a slightly bitter flavor. It helps to stimulate digestion and cleanse the liver. Serves 4.

2 bunches arugula

1 small head radicchio

1 medium cucumber, sliced in thin half rounds

1/2 small red onion, cut into paper thin slices

2 tablespoons extra virgin olive oil

1/4 cup freshly squeezed orange juice

1 teaspoon honey

1/8 teaspoon sea salt, or to taste

freshly ground black pepper

1. Wash arugula and radicchio and tear into large bite-sized pieces. Add cucumber and red onion. 2. Combine olive oil, orange juice, honey, sea salt, and black pepper. Pour over salad and mix. Adjust seasonings and serve.

Carrot Apple Salad

Grated raw carrots and apples make a sweet, cleansing salad rich in carotenoids and pectin, a soluble fiber. Serves 4.

3 cups grated carrots

1 large apple, diced

2 tablespoons currants

4 tablespoons walnuts, chopped coarsely

2 tablespoons fresh lemon juice

juice of 1 large orange

1 tablespoon grated orange peel

1 teaspoon maple syrup

1/2 teaspoon ground cinnamon

pinch of sea salt

1. Mix together grated carrots, apple, currants, and walnuts.

2. Combine fresh orange juice, lemon juice, grated orange peel, maple syrup, cinnamon, and sea salt. Pour over carrot combination and mix well. Adjust seasonings and serve.

Asparagus with Roasted Red Peppers

Asparagus is rich in glutathione, a potent antioxidant. It also has diuretic properties and helps to cleanse the kidneys. Serves 4.

1 pound fresh asparagus

1 red bell pepper, roasted, peeled, and sliced in strips

2 tablespoons extra virgin olive oil

1 tablespoon fresh lemon juice

1 teaspoon grated lemon peel

1 teaspoon dijon mustard

1 teaspoon honey

1 tablespoon minced fresh tarragon

sea salt and freshly ground black pepper to taste

1. Preheat oven to 475 degrees. Slice pepper in half lengthwise and remove stem and seeds.

2. Lay the pepper with cut sides down on a baking sheet lined with parchment paper. Roast approximately 15 minutes, until the skin turns dark and blisters. Remove from oven, put pepper into a bowl, and cover. Let sit for 10 minutes to cool, and then remove the skin. Slice into thin strips.

3. Cut asparagus diagonally into 3-inch pieces. Cook in salted water for 2 minutes, or until tender. Drain and rinse with cool water.

4. Combine olive oil, mustard, lemon juice, honey, lemon peel, tarragon, sea salt and freshly ground pepper in a jar and shake until well blended. Pour over asparagus and red pepper, adjust seasonings, and serve.

Avocado Grapefruit Salad

Avocados and grapefruit are both rich sources of glutathione, a powerful antioxidant that neutralizes harmful toxins. Sweet, pink grapefruit contrasts beautifully with creamy avocado. Serves 4.

1 large pink grapefruit

1 large ripe avocado

1 tablespoon extra virgin olive oil

1 head butter lettuce

sea salt and freshly ground black pepper

1. Peel and section the grapefruit. Cut the avocado in half and slice into 1-inch slices, then slice in half again. Gently mix the avocado and grapefruit together.

2. Wash and dry the lettuce. Keep small leaves whole, and tear larger leaves into smaller pieces. Add the grapefruit and avocado and olive oil. Season with sea salt and freshly ground black pepper, and toss gently.

Fresh Tomato, Corn and Black Bean Salad

Fiber-rich beans and corn combined with fresh tomatoes, onions, and parsley make a tasty main course salad that delivers a wealth of phytonutrients. Serves 4.

2 cups cooked black beans

1 cup cooked fresh corn

1 cup chopped ripe tomatoes

1/2 cup chopped purple onion

1/4 cup chopped fresh parsley

1/4 cup chopped fresh basil

2 tablespoons extra virgin olive oil

1 tablespoon fresh lemon juice

1/2 teaspoon sea salt

freshly ground black pepper to taste

Combine all ingredients and mix gently. Adjust seasoning by adding more lemon juice or sea salt if necessary. Chill for 1 hour to allow flavors to mingle, and serve on a bed of mixed lettuces.

Broccoli and White Bean Salad

This bean and vegetable salad is rich in soluble fibers, and offers the cancer-preventive nutrients of broccoli, onion, and red peppers. Serves 4.

2 cups broccoli florets

1 cup carrots, sliced in 1/4-inch thick half moons

1 1/2 cups cooked white beans

1/2 medium purple onion, chopped

1/2 red bell pepper, chopped

2 tablespoons finely chopped fresh basil

1/4 cup extra virgin olive oil

2 tablespoons fresh lemon juice

1 teaspoon dijon mustard

2 teaspoons honey

1/2 teaspoon sea salt, or to taste

freshly ground black pepper

1. Blanch broccoli and carrots separately in rapidly boiling salted water just until barely tender, approximately 1 minute. Remove and cool under cold running water. Drain.

2. In a large bowl, mix together white beans, purple onion, red bell pepper, and basil. Add broccoli and carrots.

3. Combine olive oil, lemon juice, mustard, honey, and sea salt. Pour over bean and vegetable mixture. Add freshly ground black pepper and mix gently. Allow to stand for at least 15 minutes before serving, and adjust seasonings.

Orange Vinaigrette

Freshly squeezed orange juice gives a refreshing, slightly sweet flavor to this vinaigrette. Grated orange rind provides the phytonutrient limonene, which helps to detoxify the liver.

4 tablespoons extra virgin olive oil

1 teaspoon honey

1 tablespoon Dijon-style mustard

1/2 cup freshly squeezed orange juice

1 tablespoon grated orange rind

1/4 teaspoon sea salt, or to taste

1/4 teaspoon freshly ground black pepper

Combine all ingredients in a small jar and shake well. Serve on mixed greens or watercress.

Creamy Tofu Dressing

Tofu adds richness to salad dressings and also provides phytoestrogens, which have cancer-preventive properties. Makes approximately 1 1/2 cups.

1 cup silken tofu

2 tablespoons light miso

2 tablespoons extra virgin olive oil

1 tablespoon fresh lemon juice

1/4 cup freshly squeezed orange juice

1 tablespoon freshly grated orange peel

2 teaspoons freshly grated ginger root

2 tablespoons minced chives

1 teaspoon honey

freshly ground black pepper to taste

2 tablespoons toasted sesame seeds

Combine all ingredients except sesame seeds in a blender or food processor and puree until smooth. Stir in sesame seeds.

Soups

Simple Vegetable Stock

A good vegetable stock adds richness and extra nutrients to soup. This basic stock can be used as the foundation for any soup recipe and can be used as a broth during a cleansing program with the addition of a bit of miso and chopped scallions.

3 stalks celery with leaves, cut into 2-inch pieces

1 medium leek, cut into 2-inch pieces

3 medium carrots, cut into 2-inch pieces

3 medium onions, quartered

1 large potato, cut into large chunks

4 garlic cloves, chopped

2-inch piece fresh ginger root, chopped

1/2 bunch fresh parsley

1/2 teaspoon sea salt

Place ingredients into a large pot. Add 10 cups of water and bring to a boil over medium heat. Reduce heat and simmer gently for 1 hour.

Strain stock through a fine strainer. Refrigerate and use stock within a couple of days or freeze and use within 3 months.

Roasted Root Vegetable Stock

Roasted root vegetables give this stock a sweet, deep flavor. Use as a base for intensely flavored soups. Add a teaspoon of miso to one cup of stock and a bit of chopped scallion and you have an instant healthful cleansing broth.

2 medium burdock roots, scrubbed and cut into 1-inch chunks

2 large parsnips, scrubbed and cut into 1-inch chunks

4 large carrots, scrubbed and cut into 1-inch chunks

2 medium onions, peeled and quartered

1 head garlic, separated into cloves

2-inch piece of ginger, sliced into 1/4-inch rounds

2 tablespoons extra virgin olive oil

1/2 teaspoon sea salt

4 dried shiitake mushrooms

1. Preheat oven to 425 degrees. Put the vegetables into a large roasting pan and mix with olive oil and sea salt. Roast for approximately 30 minutes, stirring occasionally.

2. Remove vegetables from oven and transfer to a large pot with 10 cups of water. Add shiitake mushrooms. Bring to a boil over medium heat, lower heat, and simmer covered, for 1 hour.

3. Strain through a fine mesh strainer, extracting as much liquid from the vegetables as possible. Refrigerate stock and use within a couple of days or freeze for up to 3 months.

Miso Shiitake Soup

This warming broth is excellent as a fall or winter cleansing tonic soup. Shiitake mushrooms have potent immune-enhancing properties, and miso helps to replenish healthy intestinal flora. Serves 4.

1 cup shiitake mushrooms, sliced

1 cup carrots, sliced into thin half moons

1 1/2-inch piece of ginger root, thinly sliced

2 cloves garlic, minced

2 tablespoons extra virgin olive oil

5 cups vegetable stock or water

2 tablespoons light miso, or to taste

2 scallions, cut diagonally into 2-inch pieces

1. In a heavy pot over medium heat, sauté shiitake mushrooms, carrots, and ginger, in olive oil for 3 minutes. Add garlic and sauté 1 minute.

2. Add vegetable broth or water and simmer, covered, for an additional 5 minutes, or until carrots are tender. Turn off heat.

3. Dissolve miso in a small amount of hot soup broth and stir into soup. Add scallions and cover. Let stand for 2 minutes, and serve.

Carrot Soup with Dill

This simple and delicious soup provides a potent dose of beta-carotene. Miso adds beneficial friendly flora. Serves 4.

4 cups carrots, chopped

1 cup purple onion, chopped

1 cup potato, peeled and chopped

2 tablespoons extra virgin olive oil

5 cups vegetable stock or water

2 tablespoons light miso or sea salt to taste

2 tablespoon fresh dill, minced

freshly ground black pepper to taste

1. Sauté carrots, onion, and potato in olive oil over medium heat for 5 minutes. Add vegetable stock or water and simmer for 30 minutes, or until vegetables are soft.

2. Cool slightly, and puree soup in a blender or food processor with lemon and miso. Return to soup pot and add dill and freshly ground black pepper. Heat gently and serve.

Spring Tonic Soup

This delicate and delicious soup combines leeks, asparagus, and parsley for a spring tonic cleansing soup. Serves 4.

1 small leek, sliced into thin crescents

1/2 cup shiitake mushrooms, sliced

1/2 cup carrots, sliced into 1/4-inch half moons

1-inch piece of fresh ginger root, thinly sliced

2 cloves garlic, minced

2 tablespoons extra virgin olive oil

5 cups vegetable stock or water

1 cup asparagus, cut diagonally into 1-inch pieces

2 tablespoons light miso, or to taste

1/4 cup parsley, finely minced

freshly ground black pepper

1. In a large heavy pot over medium heat, sauté leek, shiitake mushrooms, carrots, ginger root, and garlic in olive oil until vegetables have softened, approximately 5 minutes.

2. Add vegetable stock or water and bring to a boil. Lower heat, cover, and simmer for 10 minutes. Add asparagus, and simmer for an additional 5 minutes or until asparagus is tender.

3. Dilute miso in a small amount of hot broth and add to soup. Turn off heat and add parsley. Cover, and allow to stand for 5 minutes. Add freshly ground black pepper and adjust seasonings. Serve.

Autumn Tonic Soup

This soup combines the earthy root vegetables of autumn into a tasty, purifying tonic soup. Burdock is rich in minerals and is a classic liver-cleansing herb. Serves 4.

1/2 cup burdock root, scrubbed and sliced into 1/2-inch half moons

1/2 cup carrots, sliced into 1/2-inch half moons

1/2 cup cabbage, thinly sliced

1/2 cup parsnips, sliced into 1/2-inch half moons

1/2 cup red onion, chopped

1/2 cup shiitake mushrooms, sliced

3 cloves garlic, minced

2 tablespoons extra virgin olive oil

5 cups vegetable stock or water

2 tablespoons light miso, or to taste

2 scallions, minced

freshly ground black pepper

1. In a large, heavy pot over medium heat, sauté burdock, carrots, cabbage, parsnips, onion, shiitake, and garlic in olive oil for 10 minutes.

2. Add vegetable stock or water and bring to a boil. Lower heat, cover, and simmer for 20 minutes or until vegetables are tender.

3. Dilute miso in a small amount of hot broth and add to soup. Turn off heat, add scallions, cover, and let stand for 5 minutes. Season with freshly ground black pepper, if desired.

Corn Chowder

This sweet chowder is wonderful made with fresh corn. Corn is rich in fiber, and shiitake mushrooms and onions add immune-enhancing benefits. Serves 4.

1/2 cup red onion, chopped

1/2 cup red bell pepper, chopped

1/2 cup shiitake mushrooms, chopped

2 tablespoons extra virgin olive oil

2 cloves garlic, minced

1-inch fresh ginger root, thinly sliced

2 cups corn, cut off cob

5 cups vegetable stock or water

2 tablespoons light miso or sea salt to taste

1/4 cup fresh parsley or basil, minced

freshly ground black pepper

1. In a large, heavy pot over medium heat, sauté onion, red bell pepper, shiitake, garlic, and ginger in olive oil for 5 minutes.

2. Add corn and vegetable stock or water and bring to a boil. Lower heat, cover, and simmer for 15 minutes.

3. Dilute miso in a small amount of hot soup broth and add to soup. Turn off heat, add parsley or basil, cover, and let stand for 5 minutes before serving. Season with freshly ground black pepper.

Sweet Winter Squash Soup

Deep orange winter squashes are rich in carotenes. My favorites are buttercup and kabocha, which are sweeter than butternut.

4 cups buttercup or other winter squash

1 medium onion, coarsely chopped

2 tablespoons olive oil

3 cups water

1 tablespoon grated organic orange peel

2 tablespoons grated fresh ginger root

2 tablespoons light miso, or to taste

2 tablespoons parsley, finely minced

1. Peel and chop squash into 1-inch chunks.

2. In a large, heavy pot, sauté onion in olive oil until soft. Add squash and water and simmer for 30 minutes, until squash is soft. Let cool slightly, and puree in blender or food processor with miso.

3. Return to soup pot and add grated orange peel. Squeeze the juice from the grated ginger into the soup. Reheat the soup, and add parsley and freshly grated black pepper. Adjust seasonings and serve.

Main Dishes

Cabbage Tofu Rolls

Cabbage, tofu, and shiitake mushrooms make this a powerful antioxidant, phytonutrient rich main dish. Serves 4.

8 large leaves Chinese cabbage

1 medium purple onion, chopped

1 cup shiitake mushrooms, chopped

1/2 cup red bell pepper, chopped

3 cloves garlic, minced

1 teaspoon fennel seeds

2 tablespoons extra virgin olive oil

8 ounces firm tofu, drained and crumbled

2 tablespoons tamari (natural soy sauce)

2 teaspoons fresh lemon juice

1/2 cup walnuts, chopped coarsely

1/4 teaspoon dried thyme leaves, crumbled

1/4 cup fresh parsley, minced

sea salt and freshly ground black pepper to taste

1. Place tofu in a colander to drain off excess water. Blanch cabbage leaves in a large pot of boiling water for approximately 2 minutes. Set aside to cool.

2. Sauté onion, shiitake mushrooms, red bell pepper, and garlic in olive oil over medium heat until onion is translucent.

3. Add crumbled tofu, tamari, lemon juice, walnuts, thyme, and parsley and mix well. Cook until tofu is heated through. Add freshly ground black pepper and sea salt to taste.

4. Preheat oven to 350 degrees. To assemble the cabbage rolls, place approximately 1/2 cup of filling at the end of each cabbage leaf. Fold the sides toward the center over the filling, and beginning at an end, roll

the leaf up lengthwise. Secure with a toothpick if necessary. Place the rolls seam side down in a baking dish. Cover the pan tightly with foil and bake for 20 minutes.

Sautéed Tempeh with Broccoli

This quick main dish combines phytonutrient-rich tempeh with broccoli, one of the best-loved cruciferous vegetables. Serves 4.

8 ounces tempeh, chopped into 1/2-inch cubes

1/4 cup tamari (natural soy sauce)

1/4 cup water

2 teaspoons honey

4 tablespoons extra virgin olive oil

1 tablespoon grated fresh ginger root

2 cloves garlic, minced

1/2 medium purple onion, thinly sliced into half-moons

1 large red bell pepper, thinly sliced

4 cups broccoli, cut into small florets

1. Combine tamari, water, honey, ginger root, and garlic in a saucepan and bring to a boil. Lower the heat, add tempeh, and simmer, covered for 20 minutes. Remove from heat, remove lid, and allow to cool to room temperature. Remove tempeh from marinade and reserve marinade.

2. In a large skillet or wok, heat 2 tablespoons olive oil over medium heat. Add tempeh and sauté until golden. Remove tempeh.

3. Add additional 2 tablespoons of oil and sauté ginger, onion, and red pepper until onion begins to soften. Add broccoli and garlic and cook for 3 minutes. Add tempeh and marinade and cook for 1 minute, or until broccoli is tender.

Vegetable Paella

This grain and vegetable main dish offers an abundance of fiber from brown rice and chickpeas. Substitute cooked chicken, fish, or shrimp for the chickpeas if desired. Serves 3 to 4.

1 cup raw brown basmati rice

1/4 teaspoon sea salt

3 cups vegetable stock or water

2 tablespoons extra virgin olive oil

1 medium onion, chopped

2 garlic cloves, minced

1 red bell pepper, thinly sliced

1/2 teaspoon saffron threads

1 large tomato, chopped

1 cup cooked chickpeas

1 cup frozen green peas

freshly ground black pepper

fresh cilantro

1. *Cook rice in 1 1/2 cups water until liquid is absorbed.*

2. *In a heavy skillet, sauté onions, garlic, and peppers in olive oil until tender. Add rice, saffron, tomato, chickpeas, and the remaining 1 1/2 cups water. Cover and cook over low heat for 30 minutes.*

3. *Add green peas and continue cooking uncovered for another 5 minutes, until all liquid is absorbed.*

4. *Garnish with chopped cilantro and season with freshly ground black pepper.*

Tempeh with Shiitake Mushrooms

Tempeh contains potent cancer-fighting phytoestrogens, and shiitake mushrooms enhance immune functioning. Serves 4.

1 medium red onion, chopped

1 medium red bell pepper, chopped

2 cloves garlic, minced

1/2 teaspoon sea salt, or to taste

1 cup sliced shiitake mushrooms

4 tablespoons extra virgin olive oil

12 ounces tempeh, chopped finely

1/2 cup organic red wine

1/2 cup water

1/4 cup parsley, minced

freshly ground black pepper to taste

1. *Sauté onion, red bell pepper, garlic, sea salt, and shiitake mushrooms in olive oil over medium heat until onions are translucent.*

2. *Add finely chopped tempeh and stir, sautéing until tempeh turns golden.*

3. Add wine, water, parsley, and freshly ground black pepper and cook for 5 minutes. Adjust seasonings and serve over brown rice or pasta.

Marinated Grilled Tofu

Marinating tofu gives it a whole new personality. Tofu is rich in nutrients that provide potent protection against cancer. Serves 4.

1 pound firm tofu, drained

1 tablespoon extra virgin olive oil

2 tablespoons tamari (natural soy sauce)

1/4 cup freshly squeezed orange juice

1 tablespoon fresh lime juice

1 tablespoon honey

1 tablespoon freshly grated ginger root

2 cloves garlic, minced

1/4 teaspoon freshly ground black pepper

1. Place tofu in a colander for 15 minutes to drain off excess water.

2. Combine remaining ingredients and mix well.

3. Slice the tofu into 1-inch thick rectangles. Place in a shallow dish and pour marinade over the tofu pieces. Allow to marinate for at least 2 hours, flipping the tofu pieces a couple of times during the process to allow them to soak up the marinade evenly.

4. Remove from marinade and grill tofu on a grill or under the broiler until golden.

Mediterranean Fish Stew

Chunks of fresh fish combine with antioxidant rich tomatoes, onions, and garlic for a satisfying one-dish meal. Serves 4.

1 large purple onion, chopped

3 garlic cloves, minced

1 inch fresh ginger root, thinly sliced

2 teaspoons fennel seeds

2 tablespoons extra virgin olive oil

2 cups sliced fennel or celery

4 cups red potatoes, peeled and cubed

3 cups plum tomatoes, chopped

4 cups vegetable stock

1 tablespoon grated fresh orange peel

2 fresh rosemary sprigs

1/4 teaspoon saffron

1 pound firm white fish fillets, such as halibut or cod

sea salt and freshly ground black pepper to taste

fresh parsley for garnish

1. Sauté onions, garlic, ginger, and fennel seeds in olive oil in a large heavy pot over medium heat until the onions are translucent. Add a bit of water if necessary to prevent the garlic from browning.

2. Add chopped fennel or celery, potatoes, tomatoes, orange peel, rosemary, and vegetable stock. Bring to a boil, lower the heat, cover, and simmer for 20 minutes.

3. Cut fish into 1 1/2-inch chunks. Add the saffron and fish to the stew and cook for another 10 minutes, or until the fish is cooked through. Season with sea salt and freshly ground black pepper to taste and garnish with minced parsley.

Salmon with Honey Mustard Glaze on Greens

This dish can be put together quickly and makes an elegant presentation. Salmon is a rich source of omega-3 essential fatty acids. Serves 4.

4 salmon fillets, 6 ounces each

1 1/2 tablespoons honey

1 1/2 tablespoons dijon mustard

2 teaspoons extra virgin olive oil

2 tablespoons fresh orange juice

1/4 teaspoon sea salt

freshly ground black pepper

1 large bunch mustard greens

1. Preheat oven to 400 degrees. Rinse and pat salmon fillets dry. Place in a single layer in an ovenproof baking dish.

2. Mix together honey, mustard, olive oil, orange juice, and sea salt. Spread over salmon fillets. Bake for 15 minutes, or until fish flakes easily with a fork.

3. Wash mustard greens, remove stems, and slice into 2-inch wide strips. Bring 2 cups of salted water to boil in a large pot and cook mustard greens for 3 minutes, or until tender. Remove with slotted spoon and drain.

4. To serve, divide mustard greens among four plates and top with cooked salmon fillets.

Vegetable and Grain Side Dishes

Quick Cooked Greens

Cultivate the habit of eating dark leafy greens daily. Their slightly bitter flavor stimulates liver function. Quick boiling greens preserves more nutrients than steaming and results in better flavor. Serves 4.

1 bunch of greens, such as kale, collards, or mustard

1/4 teaspoon sea salt

1. Wash greens. Remove tough stems and center ribs, and slice greens crosswise.

2. Bring 2 cups of water and 1/4 teaspoon of sea salt to a boil in a large pot. Add greens, cover, and cook over high heat for approximately 5 minutes, or until tender. Drain and serve.

Sautéed Greens with Garlic

Sautéed greens are quick to prepare and a tasty alternative to steamed greens. Greens are rich in chlorophyll, carotenoids, and calcium. Serves 4.

1 large bunch greens, such as dandelion, kale, or mustard greens

1 tablespoon extra virgin olive oil

2 garlic cloves, minced

sea salt, lemon, and freshly ground black pepper to taste

1. Blanch greens quickly in boiling water for 1 minute. Drain and chop coarsely.

2. Sauté garlic in olive oil for 30 seconds. Add greens and sea salt and toss to coat with olive oil. Sauté for 2 minutes, or until tender. Season to taste with sea salt, lemon, and freshly ground black pepper.

Kale with Currants and Pumpkin Seeds

This is a delicious way to get your daily greens. Serves 4.

1 large bunch kale

1 tablespoon extra virgin olive oil

1-inch piece of ginger root, peeled and finely chopped

1/4 cup toasted pumpkin seeds

1/4 cup currants

sea salt

1. *Toast pumpkin seeds in a heavy skillet, stirring constantly until golden.*

2. *Blanch kale quickly in boiling salted water for 1 minute. Drain and chop coarsely.*

3. *Sauté ginger in olive oil in a skillet over medium heat for 1 minute, or until golden. Add currants and greens and cook until greens are tender. Season with sea salt, black pepper, and lemon to taste. Add toasted pumpkin seeds and serve.*

Spinach with Sesame Seeds

Spinach is a good source of carotenes and chlorophyll. Toasted sesame seeds add a satisfying crunch and are rich in calcium. Serves 4.

2 tablespoons unhulled sesame seeds

2 bunches fresh spinach

1 tablespoon tamari (natural soy sauce)

1 tablespoon extra virgin olive oil

1 teaspoon honey

1. *Toast sesame seeds in a heavy skillet over medium heat for several minutes until they turn golden. Remove from pan to cool.*

2. *Wash spinach and remove stems. Place in a large pot over high heat and steam spinach for 2 minutes, or until tender. No extra water other than the water clinging to the leaves from washing should be needed to steam the spinach.*

3. *Mix together tamari, olive oil, honey, and sesame seeds and pour over the spinach. Toss to coat evenly and serve.*

Garlic Mashed Potatoes

This is an easy and delicious way to get a healthy portion of garlic. Parsley adds a pleasing contrast and plenty of chlorophyll. Yellow Finn or Yukon Gold are the tastiest potatoes to use. Serves 4.

4 cups peeled and cubed potatoes

12 garlic cloves, peeled

2 tablespoons extra virgin olive oil

sea salt and freshly ground black pepper to taste

4 tablespoons fresh parsley, finely chopped

1. Place potatoes and garlic into a pot and add just enough water to cover. Add 1/2 teaspoon sea salt and bring to a boil. Lower the heat, cover, and simmer for 15 minutes, until the potatoes are tender. Drain, reserving the cooking liquid.

2. Mash the potatoes and garlic with olive oil. Mix in reserved cooking liquid, a small amount at a time, to achieve a fluffy texture. Add parsley, sea salt, and freshly ground black pepper to taste.

Red Peppers Stuffed with Rice, Corn, and Basil

Red bell peppers are a rich source of carotenes, and brown rice and corn are high in cleansing fiber. This makes a colorful vegetable side dish. Serves 4.

2 cups cooked basmati brown rice

2 tablespoons extra virgin olive oil

1 medium purple onion, finely chopped

2 garlic cloves, minced

1 stalk celery, finely chopped

1/2 cup fresh corn

1/2 cup pine nuts, lightly toasted

2 tablespoons fresh basil, finely chopped

sea salt and freshly ground black pepper

4 medium red bell peppers

1. Preheat oven to 375 degrees. Sauté onion, garlic, celery, and corn in olive oil until onion is soft. Add pine nuts, basil, and rice and season with sea salt and freshly ground black pepper.

2. Cut tops off peppers and remove seeds and inner membranes. Cut a thin slice off the bottom of each pepper to allow it to stand on end.

3. Pack the peppers lightly with the rice and vegetable mixture, and place them into a baking dish just large enough to hold them upright. Drizzle a bit of olive oil over the top of each pepper. Add 1 inch of water to the baking dish.

4. Bake, uncovered, for approximately 1 hour, or until peppers are soft when pierced with a knife. Serve.

Grilled Vegetable Kebabs

Grill these kebabs outdoors or broil them indoors. Shiitake mushrooms are meaty and flavorful and contain powerful immune-enhancing compounds. Serves 6.

12 shiitake mushrooms

1 large red pepper, cut into 1-inch squares

12 cherry tomatoes

3 scallions, cut into 2-inch pieces

2 small zucchini, cut into 1/2-inch rounds

2 small yellow squash, cut into 1/2-inch rounds

Marinade:

2 tablespoons extra virgin olive oil

1/4 cup tamari (natural soy sauce)

1/2 cup water

2 tablespoons lemon juice

1 teaspoon honey

3 cloves garlic, minced

3 tablespoons minced tarragon

freshly ground black pepper

1. Combine marinade ingredients and add cut up vegetables. Marinate for 2 hours or longer, stirring occasionally to coat all of the vegetables with the marinade.

2. Skewer vegetables on bamboo kebab sticks, and place kebabs on a hot grill or in a baking dish under the broiler. Cook for 5 minutes on each side until vegetables are cooked through.

Quinoa with Corn

Quinoa is a quick-cooking mineral rich grain that makes a fluffy pilaf. This is a terrific side dish with fish, chicken, or grilled tofu. Serves 4.

1 cup quinoa

2 tablespoons extra virgin olive oil

1/2 medium red onion, finely chopped

1/2 red bell pepper, finely chopped

2 cloves garlic, minced

2 cups vegetable stock or water

1 cup fresh corn kernels

1/2 teaspoon sea salt

1/4 cup fresh parsley, minced

freshly ground black pepper

1. Rinse quinoa thoroughly and drain.

2. In a heavy pot over medium heat, sauté onion, red bell pepper, and garlic in olive oil for 2 minutes. Add quinoa and 2 cups of vegetable stock or water, corn, and salt. Bring to a boil, cover, reduce heat, and simmer for 15 minutes.

3. Turn off heat and add parsley. Let sit, covered, for 5 minutes. Add freshly ground black pepper, fluff quinoa with a fork, and serve.

Asparagus with Lemon

Enjoy asparagus often during the few weeks that it is in season. Asparagus is a wonderful, spring cleansing vegetable. Serves 4.

1 pound asparagus

2 tablespoons extra virgin olive oil

4 cloves garlic, minced

1 lemon, juiced

1 teaspoon finely grated lemon peel

sea salt and freshly ground black pepper to taste

1. Cook asparagus spears in boiling water until tender, approximately 3-4 minutes. Drain.

2. Heat olive oil in a skillet over medium heat, add garlic, and sauté for 1 minute, being careful to not burn the garlic. Add the lemon peel, black pepper, sea salt, and lemon juice and cook for 1 minute. Toss with asparagus and serve.

Accompaniments

Onion and Red Pepper Confit

This savory and sweet confit is delicious with fish, chicken, or bean dishes. Onions are rich in quercetin, a potent antioxidant.

2 tablespoons extra virgin olive oil

2 large purple onions, sliced into 1/4-inch half moons

3 garlic cloves, minced

2 large red bell peppers, sliced into 1/4-inch strips

1 tablespoon fresh thyme or oregano leaves

sea salt and freshly ground black pepper

1. Heat olive oil in a large, heavy skillet over medium heat. Add onions and a pinch of sea salt and sauté approximately 10 minutes, stirring frequently until they turn translucent.

2. Add peppers, garlic, and thyme or oregano and lower heat. Cover, and cook for approximately 45 minutes, until the onions are soft and golden and the peppers are soft.

3. Season to taste with sea salt and freshly ground black pepper. Remove from heat and cool. Refrigerate for up to 3 days.

Mango Salsa

This is a wonderful accompaniment to grilled salmon or chicken. Mangoes are rich in carotenes. Serves 4.

1 ripe mango, pitted, peeled, and diced

1/2 red bell pepper, diced

1/2 purple onion, diced

1/2 small jicama, diced

1/4 cup cilantro, minced

juice from 1 lime

sea salt and freshly ground black pepper

Mix all ingredients together and season to taste with sea salt and freshly ground black pepper.

Salsa Fresca

This simple salsa is a good accompaniment for fish, chicken, or bean dishes. Tomatoes are high in lycopene, a potent antioxidant. Makes approximately 4 cups.

1 pound ripe tomatoes, cored and chopped

1/2 medium purple onion, minced

1/2 cup cilantro, minced

juice of 1 lime (approximately 1/4 cup)

sea salt and freshly ground black pepper to taste

Combine all ingredients and season with sea salt and freshly ground black pepper.

Tofu Basil Dip

This dip can be thinned with water to make a sauce for grains or vegetables. Tofu is an excellent source of phytoestrogens, which have natural anticancer properties.

1 pound firm tofu

1 bunch fresh basil

1/4 cup extra virgin olive oil

1/4 cup water

1 tablespoon lemon juice

2 cloves fresh garlic

1 teaspoon honey

2 tablespoon light miso

freshly ground black pepper

1. Cook tofu in boiling water for 5 minutes. Remove from heat and place in cold water to cool.

2. Puree basil, water, and olive oil in blender on low speed for 1 minute. Add lemon juice, garlic, honey, and miso and blend until smooth. Season with freshly ground black pepper to taste and adjust seasonings.

Guacamole with Fresh Tomatoes and Cilantro

Avocados provide a healthy dose of glutathione, a natural antioxidant. Fresh tomatoes lighten it up and offer lycopene, another potent antioxidant. Makes approximately 2 cups.

2 large ripe avocados

1/4 cup fresh lemon juice

1/2 teaspoon sea salt, or to taste

1 medium tomato, finely chopped

1/2 small red onion, finely chopped

1 small fresh chile, seeded and minced

1 tablespoon fresh cilantro, finely minced

1. Slice the avocados in half lengthwise and remove the pits. Scoop out the avocado flesh with a spoon into a bowl. Mash with lemon juice and salt.

2. Add tomato, red onion, chile, and cilantro and mix well. Adjust seasonings and serve.

Hummus with Parsley

Grated lemon peel, parsley, and scallions make this a lively tasting hummus and provide beneficial phytonutrients. Sesame tahini is rich in calcium. Makes approximately 2 1/2 cups.

3 cups cooked chickpeas, drained (reserve cooking water)

2 tablespoons sesame tahini

2 tablespoons extra virgin olive oil

1/4 cup fresh lemon juice

1/4 cup chickpea cooking liquid or water

2 cloves garlic, minced

2 scallions, minced

2 teaspoons grated lemon peel

1/3 cup parsley, minced

1 teaspoon sea salt

freshly ground black pepper

1. Place all ingredients in a blender or food processor and puree until smooth.

2. Adjust seasoning by adding more lemon juice, sea salt, or freshly ground black pepper if necessary.

Tahini-Orange Sauce

This sauce is delicious over steamed broccoli or whole grains. Tahini is rich in calcium, and grated orange rind adds the cancer-preventive power of limonene.

2 tablespoons unhulled sesame seeds, toasted

1/2 cup sesame tahini

2 tablespoons honey

3 tablespoons tamari (natural soy sauce)

1 tablespoon lemon juice

1/2 cup freshly squeezed orange juice

2 scallions, minced

1 tablespoon finely grated orange peel

1. Toast sesame seeds in a heavy skillet over medium heat until golden and fragrant. Set aside to cool.

2. Combine tahini, honey, tamari, and lemon juice in a bowl and mix until well blended. Add the orange juice a little at a time and blend until creamy. Stir in the scallions and grated orange peel. Serve over steamed vegetables or whole grains.

Desserts

Gingered Fruit Compote

This compote is a simple dessert or a nice breakfast beginning. It has gentle laxative properties. Yields four cups.

1 pound assorted dried prunes, currants, apricots, and apples

1 stick cinnamon

1-inch piece fresh ginger root, sliced thinly

pinch sea salt

1. Place ingredients in a saucepan and add enough water to just cover the fruit. Simmer, covered, over low heat for 1 hour, stirring occasionally.

2. Keep refrigerated for up to 1 week.

Peaches in Strawberry Sauce

This is a summertime dessert treat and a beautiful contrast of colors. Peaches and strawberries are good sources of vitamin C, and strawberries contain ellagic acid, a cancer-preventive nutrient. Serves 4.

4 large ripe peaches, sliced

1 pint strawberries

1 tablespoon maple syrup

2 tablespoons almonds, toasted and chopped

fresh mint

1. Puree strawberries and maple syrup in a blender.

2. Arrange peaches in a glass bowl, and pour strawberry sauce over the peaches. Garnish with toasted almonds and whole fresh mint leaves.

Apples Poached with Cinnamon and Vanilla

Poached apples are delicious for either breakfast or as a dessert. Apples are rich in pectin, a soluble fiber. Serves 4.

5 cups apple juice

2 cinnamon sticks

1/2 vanilla bean

4 firm apples

1. *Combine apple juice, cinnamon sticks, and vanilla bean in a pot large enough to hold apples in a single layer.*

2. *Peel and core apples and add to liquid. Add additional apple juice if necessary to cover the apples. Bring to a simmer over medium heat, and cook gently until apples are just tender, approximately 10 minutes.*

3. *Remove apples from poaching liquid and place in a large bowl. Remove cinnamon sticks and vanilla bean and reduce poaching liquid to a syrup by simmering uncovered for approximately 30 minutes. Pour over apples and cool to room temperature. Chill before serving.*

4. *To serve, place in dessert bowls and spoon syrup over apples. Garnish with fresh mint leaves.*

chapter fourteen

Exercise to Increase Detoxification

*E*xercise is essential for the process of detoxification. Physical activity increases respiratory and circulatory function, stimulates lymphatic flow, improves digestive function and elimination, strengthens the immune system, improves sleep quality, and may be the most effective treatment for relieving anxiety and depression.

Your body needs daily exercise to stay healthy and strong. If you are already exercising regularly, you are most likely well aware of the many benefits you are receiving. If you're not yet in the habit of exercising, a cleansing program provides a perfect opportunity to begin enjoying the positive aspects of exercise.

To help your body detoxify, incorporate aerobic activities and stretching exercises into your daily life. Aerobic activities strengthen the cardiovascular system and enhance circulation, improve lung capacity, oxygenate the cells, and increase the elimination of toxins. Stretching exercises such as yoga increase flexibility, calm the nervous system, and provide an internal massage which improves the health of all organs and glands.

The Cleansing Benefits of Aerobic Exercise

Everyone knows that aerobic exercise is good for the cardiovascular system. But the health-enhancing benefits of aerobic exercise go far beyond just strengthening your heart muscle. Aerobic exercise is one of the best ways to oxygenate your cells. Without regular exercise, waste materials accumulate in the tissues and organs, resulting in degenerative disease and premature aging. Aerobic activity increases the heart rate, speeds up circulation, and expands lung capacity, which sends fresh oxygenated blood coursing through your body to nourish and purify your organs. The lymphatic system cleanses all of the cells, and relies on the rhythmical contractions of muscles during exercise to move lymph through the body. Exercise also improves the functioning of the digestive organs and stimulates peristalsis to help move wastes out of the body.

CLEANSING BENEFITS OF AEROBIC EXERCISE

Improves circulation

Oxygenates cells

Increases lung capacity

Stimulates lymphatic flow

Improves digestive function

Enhances immune activity

Promotes perspiration

Stimulates peristalsis

Making Exercise Fun

The best aerobic activities are those which you enjoy doing. Think of your exercise as playtime. Vary your activities, try new ones, and find friends who also like to be active. My favorite daily exercise is an hour-long early morning hike in the hills around my home. I have cultivated at least a half-dozen walking buddies, and I schedule walking dates with a different friend each morning. It's a wonderful opportunity to socialize and I usually find that the hour passes by all too quickly! Walking is perhaps the easiest exercise for most people. It doesn't require any particular skills or any special equipment other than a pair of comfortable, supportive shoes. Swimming, bicycling, hiking, dancing, tennis, and active gardening are other good aerobic choices. For an activity to provide aerobic benefits, it needs to increase your heart rate. A longer period of sustained activity is healthier for your body than intense bursts of exercise. There's no need for complicated formulas for figuring out your heart rate and you don't need to check your pulse. Just make sure that you're exercising briskly enough so that your breathing is slightly increased and you'll be getting aerobic benefits. Exercise should make you feel good, not wear you out!

AEROBIC ACTIVITIES

Walking

Hiking

Swimming

Bicycling

Dancing

Gardening

Skiing

Tennis

Jogging

Skating

Enhancing the Benefits of Aerobic Activity

While 30 minutes of aerobic activity 3 times a week is said by many experts to be sufficient, I recommend 30 minutes or more at least 6 times a week. Your body was designed to be active, and not just for 30 minutes 3 times a week! The more you keep your energy flowing, the better you will feel. Ideally, build exercise into your life so that you are active as much as possible throughout the day. Look for opportunities to move and stretch and to enjoy your wonderful body.

To enhance the benefits of aerobic activity, pay attention to your body while you are exercising. Breathe deeply and allow healing oxygen to flow throughout your body. Focus on breathing abdominally, allowing your abdomen to expand with each inhalation, and to contract with each exhalation. Avoid shallow, upper chest only breathing, which will leave you feeling fatigued and anxious. I check in with my body periodically while I'm walking to make sure that my spine is comfortably erect, my shoulders are relaxed, and my breathing is deep and easy. I do a quick body scan, looking for any areas of tension, and when I find a tense spot, I consciously breathe into that place to help it to relax. I often go for walks in the afternoon or evening to unwind after a long day, and spend the entire time in silence, checking in with my body, scanning for any areas of tension, and sending healing energy to those places that feel tight or uncomfortable. I focus on my breathing and imagine that each inhalation is purifying my body, and that each exhalation is carrying away physical and mental toxins.

Using Your Mind to Change Your Body

Regular exercise will not only improve your health, but will also help you to look better. Exercise enhances metabolic function, tones and sculpts muscles, and stimulates the body to release excess weight. Exercise also helps to improve your posture by enhancing your awareness of your physical being. By increasing circulation and the elimination of toxins, exercise benefits skin tone and texture, too. And regular exercise engenders a sense of inner calm that radiates externally as natural beauty and vitality.

To enhance the many benefits of exercise, learn to use the power of your mind to support your body in any changes that you would like to manifest. Begin to view your body with love, and become aware of any statements of self-criticism. The part of your body that you most dislike is the part that most needs your love. When you turn your attention toward your body in a positive way, you free up energy blocks that manifest as excess weight, tension, or pain. Send love and healing energy into any part of your body that you are critical of, and focus on how much you appreciate your incredible body and the gift that it gives you by providing a home for your mind and spirit. Practice breathing fully into every part of your body, finding the places where your energy is stuck, and send healing, loving thoughts to that area.

Stretch to Purify and Renew Your Body

Stretching is also an essential component of a purification program. Not only does stretching feel good, but it helps to cleanse your tissues and organs by relieving the energy blocks caused by physical and emotional stressors. Your body naturally wants to stretch, so take a few minutes first thing in the morning to wake up with a couple of stretches, or in the evening to release any tension that you may have accumulated throughout the day. Stretching exercises can also be integrated into your day to prevent tension from building up and as a way of helping you stay attuned to your body's needs. My work often requires that I sit at a computer writing for many hours at a time. I take a break every hour for 5 minutes to perform a few of the following stretches, and find that I stay alert, refreshed, and relaxed while working. In addition, these stretches are excellent warm-ups before engaging in aerobic exercise, or as a prelude to a concentrated yoga session to prepare your body for more intense movement.

Remember to keep breathing while you are stretching, to facilitate the flow of energy throughout your body.

Energizing Stretches

Swinging Twists
*Swinging Twists loosen the spine and relieve tension
and energy blocks.*

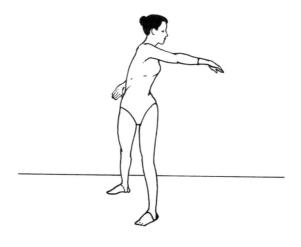

↝ Stand with your feet comfortably hip-width apart, with toes pointed straight ahead. Relax your knees slightly.

↝ With a gentle twisting motion that begins in your hips, twist your torso from side to side. Let your arms swing naturally with your body movement.

↝ Allow your head to follow the direction of your swinging arms.

Chest Expander
The Chest Expander opens the lungs and helps to relieve shoulder and upper back tension.

↝ Stand with your spine comfortably straight and your feet hip-width apart. Interlock your fingers behind your lower back, resting your hands on your buttocks.

↝ Inhale, and raise your arms behind you as far as you comfortably can. Keep your shoulders relaxed.

↝ Exhale, and lower your arms back to your buttocks. Repeat several times.

Half-Moon Pose
The Half-Moon pose opens the ribcage and provides a satisfying stretch along the sides of the body.

↝ Stand with your spine straight and your feet hip-width apart. Inhale, raise your arms straight overhead, and interlace your fingers.

↝ Exhale, and bending from your waist, slowly stretch to your right side as far as you can. Inhale, and return to center.

↝ Exhale, and bending from your waist, stretch to your left side as far as you can. Inhale, and return to center. Repeat 3 times to each side.

Shoulder Rolls
These gentle Shoulder Rolls loosen and relax the shoulders and upper back.

↝ Stand or sit in a comfortable position.

↝ Rotate your shoulders backwards, making large, smooth circles. Make 5 full circles, and then circle your shoulders forward 5 full rotations.

↝ Remember to breathe, inhaling as your shoulders come up, and exhaling as they come down.

Neck Stretches
These stretches relieve tension in the neck and help to keep the neck flexible.

- Sit or stand comfortably with your spine straight.
- Allow your head to drop forward, bringing your chin to your chest. Hold for 5-10 seconds.
- Smoothly lift your head, and allow it to gently drop back, as far as is comfortable. Hold for 5-10 seconds.
- Repeat this sequence 2 or more times, and bring your head back to center.
- Drop your right ear toward your right shoulder as far as is comfortable.

  Allow the weight of your head to pull your ear toward your shoulder.

  Hold for 5-10 seconds.
- Drop your left ear toward your left shoulder as far as is comfortable.

  Hold for 5-10 seconds.
- Repeat to each side, and return to center.

Cat Stretch
The Cat Stretch loosens the spine and relieves tension in the back and shoulders.

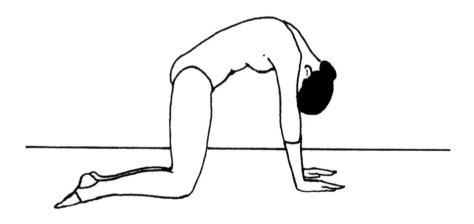

↬ Kneel down onto your hands and knees. Position your knees directly under your hips. Place your hands directly under your shoulders, with your fingers pointing forward.

↬ Exhale and curl your spine, lifting your back toward the ceiling. Tuck your chin toward your chest, and straighten your elbows to get the maximum stretch.

↬ Inhale, and relax your spine. Allow your lower back to sink gently toward the floor. Pull your shoulders down and stretch your head and neck toward the ceiling.

↬ Repeat several times.

Spinal Rocking
Gentle rocking movements relieve tension in the spine and invigorate the entire body.

↬ Sit on the floor with your knees drawn up to your chest and clasp your hands behind your knees.

↬ Round your spine slightly and tuck your chin into your chest. Gently roll backward as far as you comfortably can and then roll forward into a seated position.

↬ Continue rocking back and forth several times to loosen your spine, inhaling when you rock backward, and exhaling when you rock forward.

Rejuvenating Yoga Postures

The ancient art of hatha yoga heals the body, mind, and spirit through gentle stretching movements. Yoga is especially helpful during a cleansing program because it stimulates circulation and lymphatic flow. The twisting, bending, and stretching movements of yoga massage all the internal organs, enhancing purification and rejuvenation. Even15 minutes of daily yoga practice provides significant health benefits.

Sun Salutation
If you have time for only a few minutes of yoga, practice the Sun Salutation. This graceful series of movements stretches and rejuvenates your entire body.

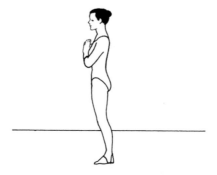

⮷ Stand with your spine straight and your feet together.
Place your palms in front of your chest in a prayer position, relax, and exhale.

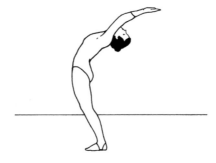

⮷ Inhale, and stretch your arms up and above your head.
Bend backwards as far as you comfortably can.

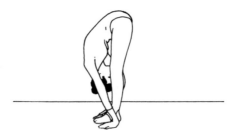

⮷ Exhale, and stretch forward, folding your body at the waist.
Bring your forehead close to your knees, keeping your legs straight but not rigid.

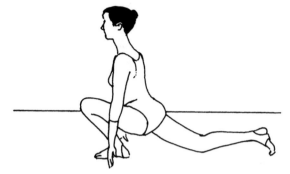

🖎 Inhale, and move your right foot back with your knee touching the floor. Place your fingertips or palms on either side of your left foot. Arch your back gently and look up.

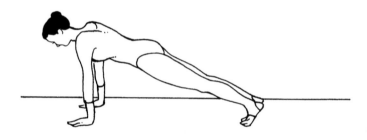

🖎 Exhale, and move your left foot back to meet your right foot. Keep your arms straight and your back and head in a straight line.

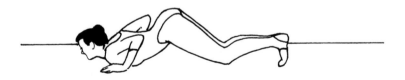

🖎 Inhale, and as you exhale, lower your body to the floor, keeping your hips and abdomen raised. Your toes, knees, chest, and hands should be resting on the floor.

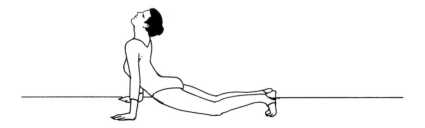

～ Inhale. Straighten your arms and gently arch your back, looking up toward the ceiling.

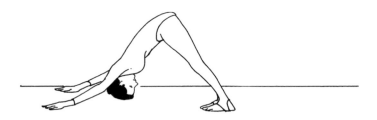

～ Exhale. Place your feet flat on the floor, and lift your hips to form a triangle position. Keep your head down and your arms and legs straight.

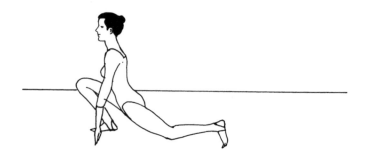

～ Inhale, and bring your right foot forward between your hands. Lower your left knee to the floor. Arch your back gently and look up.

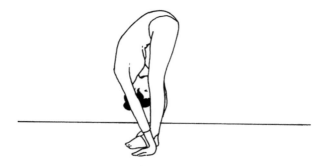

〜 Exhale, and bring your left foot forward to meet your right. Straighten your knees and bend forward from your waist. Bring your head toward your knees.

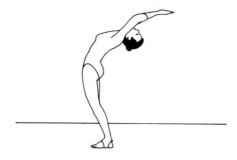

〜 Inhale, and stretch your arms over your head. Bend backward gently as far as you comfortably can.

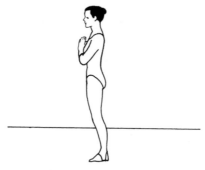

〜 Exhale. Return to standing, with your palms in prayer position in front of your chest. Repeat the sequence, this time beginning with your left leg.

Half-Locust
The Half-Locust increases circulation to the kidneys, strengthens the lower back, and stimulates large intestine function.

- Lie on your stomach with your legs extended. Point your toes away from your body. Place your chin on the floor.
- Place your arms alongside your body with your palms on the floor.
- Inhale, and stretch your right leg straight out behind your body and lift it at the same time. Keep your body straight, and don't roll onto your left side.
- Exhale, and lower your leg. Repeat to the left side.

Boat Pose
The Boat Pose strengthens the lower back and brings a fresh supply of blood to the kidneys. Do not practice this pose after the first trimester of pregnancy.

- Lie on your stomach and extend your arms straight out in front of you on the floor.
- Inhale, and raise your arms up as high as you can while at the same time raising your legs up as high as you comfortably can. Stretch and lengthen your entire body. Keep your neck relaxed. Hold for 5-10 seconds. Exhale, and relax.
- Inhale, and reach your arms straight out to the sides, lifting your upper body and your legs off the floor as high as you comfortably can. Hold for 5-10 seconds. Exhale, and relax.

The Cobra
The Cobra increases circulation to the kidneys, massages all of the abdominal organs, and helps to relieve constipation. Do not practice this pose after the first trimester of pregnancy.

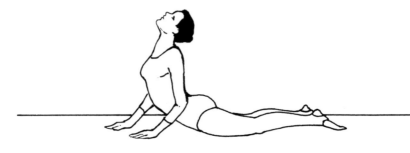

- Lie on your stomach with your forehead on the floor and your palms flat on the floor beneath your shoulders. Straighten your legs, place your feet together, and point your toes away from your body.

- Inhale, and slowly raise your head, shoulders, and upper body from the floor, using the muscles of your back. Make your movement smooth and graceful, and do not push up with your hands.

- When you have raised your body up as far as you can using only the strength of your back muscles, use your arms to lift your upper body just a bit further. Keep your elbows slightly bent, and your shoulders rolled back and down.

- Keep your abdomen on the floor and tighten your buttocks to avoid compressing your lower back. Lengthen your neck and spine, and raise your eyes to the ceiling.

- Hold the pose for 30 seconds or as long as you comfortably can, and then slowly and with control, lower your body to the floor. Bring your arms to your sides, turn your head to one side, and rest.

The Bow

The Bow massages the abdominal organs and stimulates digestion and elimination. It also brings increased circulation to the kidneys.

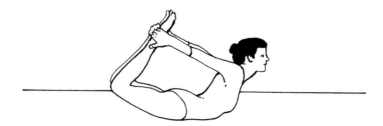

- Lie on your stomach with your arms at your sides. Bend your knees, bringing your feet toward your buttocks, and grasp your ankles.

- Inhale, contract your buttocks, and lift your head and upper body off the floor at the same time you lift your thighs off the floor. Use the strength of your arms pulling against your ankles to help to lift your body off the floor.

- Balance on your abdomen and breathe normally. Hold the pose for 30 seconds, or as long as you comfortably can.

- Slowly lower your body and release your legs.

Child Pose
This relaxing pose is a good counterbalance to back-bending poses such as the Cobra and Bow. It eases tension in the back and spine.

- ✍ Kneel on the floor, sitting on your heels with your feet and knees close together.
- ✍ Bend forward from your hips, and rest your upper body comfortably on your knees. Extend your arms straight out in front of you or place your arms beside your legs with your hands next to your feet and your palms facing upward. Rest, and breathe normally for 30 seconds or longer.

Head to Knee Pose
This pose tones the abdominal organs, stretches the spine and hamstrings, and is calming for the nervous system.

- ✍ Sit on the floor with your legs straight out in front of you. Fold your right leg and place your foot against the inside of your left thigh.
- ✍ Inhale, and reach up toward the ceiling to lengthen your spine.
- ✍ Exhale, and fold forward over your outstretched leg. Avoid rounding your back, and concentrate on lengthening your spine and bringing your abdomen toward your thigh.
- ✍ Clasp your calf, ankle, or foot. Keep your leg straight, and gently pull your body close to your leg with your arms.
- ✍ Hold the stretch for 30 seconds or as long as you comfortably can, and return to the beginning position. Repeat to the left side.

Seated Forward Bend
This pose increases circulation to the abdominal organs and stretches the entire back of the body.

- ✍ Sit on the floor with your legs straight out in front of you. Inhale, and reach your arms overhead, lengthening your spine and creating space between your vertebrae.
- ✍ Exhale, and stretch forward from your hips, reaching your arms straight out in front of your body.
- ✍ Clasp your knees, calves, or ankles. Without rounding your back, pull your upper body toward your legs by bending your elbows.

Hold for 30 seconds or as long as is comfortable, breathing slowly and deeply.

⮑ Inhale, and slowly return to a sitting position.

Shoulder stand

The Shoulder stand helps to regulate thyroid function and improves circulation. It also stimulates the digestive organs. Do not attempt the Shoulder stand if you have high blood pressure, glaucoma or other serious eye disorders, or neck problems.

⮑ Lie flat on your back with your legs straight and your feet together. Place your arms at your sides with your palms flat on the floor.

⮑ Lift your legs toward the ceiling, keeping your feet together. Place your hands behind your middle back, and raise your hips up into a 45 degree angle to the floor. Support your body with your hands, keeping your elbows and upper arms flat on the floor. Do not place weight on your neck or head. Breathe normally.

⮑ If you are comfortable in this position, straighten your body so that it is perpendicular to the floor. Tuck your chin into your chest. Your weight should be supported by your shoulders and upper arms. Do not place weight on your neck or head.

⮑ Hold for 30 seconds or as long as you comfortably can. Come out of the posture by lowering your knees to your forehead, keeping your legs straight, and rolling down one vertebra at a time until you are again lying flat on the floor.

The Fish

The Fish pose acts as a counterbalance to the Shoulderstand by arching the neck and loosening the shoulders.

⮑ Lie flat on the floor with your legs straight out in front of you and with your arms at your sides.

⮑ Arch your back, and place your hands underneath your hips. Gently slide your head back until the crown of your head is resting on the floor. Relax, and breathe deeply and slowly. Hold the posture for 30 seconds.

⮑ Slowly return to lying flat on the floor.

Spinal Twist
The Spinal Twist tones and strengthens the spine and massages the abdominal organs.

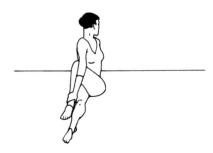

- Sit on the floor with your legs straight out in front of you.
- Cross your right leg over your left, placing your right foot on the floor to the outside of your left knee.
- Sit up straight, and twist to the right as far as you comfortably can without straining.
- Place your right hand on the floor behind you, and place your left arm on the outside of your right leg.
- Turning from your navel, twist your spine, shoulders, neck and head to look over your right shoulder. Keep your spine straight and in alignment and do not strain in this pose. Hold for 30 seconds, or as long as you comfortably can.
- Gently unwind, and return to the beginning position. Repeat to the opposite side.

The Sponge
Always end your yoga practice with at least a few minutes of this deeply relaxing and restorative pose.

- Lie flat on your back with your legs a comfortable distance apart. Place your arms next to your body with your palms facing up.
- Close your eyes, and scan your body for any areas of tension. Consciously relax those areas.
- Use your breath to help you relax. With each inhalation, imagine that you are breathing in relaxation. With each exhalation, imagine that you are breathing out tension.
- Remain in this pose for at least several minutes or for as long as you choose to.

chapter fifteen

The Healing Benefits of Hydrotherapy

*H*erbal and mineral baths, saunas, and luxurious skin-renewing treatments are a delightful indulgence and an essential component of a detoxification and purification program. Not only do these therapies wash away surface perspiration, toxins, and dead skin cells, but they also stimulate processes of deep inner cleansing to renew and refresh the body, mind, and spirit.

Hydrotherapy has been used for purification and rejuvenation by peoples all around the world, from the elaborate bathhouses of the ancient Greeks and Romans, to the hot mineral tubs of Japan and the sweat lodges of native American tribes. Natural mineral springs are considered sacred gifts from the earth and special places of healing by many traditional cultures. From earliest times until today, health seekers have made pilgrimages to mineral springs for detoxification and to relieve a wide variety of health complaints, including eczema and other skin problems, arthritis, and nervous and digestive disorders.

Many of the world's best known health spas are located at such springs, and people journey from far away to soak in the healing waters. If you have mineral baths nearby, take advantage of them as often as possible. Treat yourself once a week to a healing soak or go for a couple of days each month to enjoy the benefits of the waters. Even simpler, with the suggestions in this chapter you can create a variety of special mineral baths at home.

Adding herbs and aromatherapy essential oils can further increase the cleansing benefits of therapeutic baths. The skin is like a sponge, and readily absorbs the healing and detoxifying properties of herbs and essential oils. You can greatly enhance your cleansing program with the regular use of purifying baths and other simple water therapies. Enjoy these baths once a week for relaxation and to maintain optimal health. While undergoing a more intensive herbal cleansing program, you can soak in a mineral or herbal bath as often as every other day if desired.

Other forms of hydrotherapy that you can easily use at home include alternating hot and cold water therapy, foot baths, and sitz baths. Saunas and steams are the most powerful method of detoxification used in hydrotherapy, and are even prescribed as an essential component of medical detoxification programs for people who have been exposed to dangerous toxins. Try to use a sauna or steam bath once or twice a week during a purification program. For most people, taking a sauna once or twice a month is an excellent health habit to cultivate.

If you are pregnant, or have high blood pressure, cardiovascular disease, diabetes, circulatory disorders, or other serious health problems, do not use saunas, steams, or hot baths without the consent of your health practitioner.

Guidelines for Hydrotherapy Treatments

Hydrotherapy treatments help to purify and rejuvenate the body in a variety of ways. They stimulate increased circulation and lymphatic flow, relieve congestion throughout the body, and increase metabolism. Hot baths, saunas, and steams enhance detoxification by increasing perspiration, and are highly beneficial when used as part of a purification program. If used too frequently, though, heat treatments can cause fatigue. Use hot baths no more than 3 times a week during a cleansing program, and no more than once a week on a regular basis. Because hot baths produce a sedative effect, they are best used just before going to bed for the night. Make the water as hot as you can tolerate, but not so hot that you burn your skin or become dizzy or uncomfortable. Most people can tolerate foot baths a few degrees hotter than full baths. In general, keep hot full body baths in the range of 100 to 103 degrees, and hot foot baths between 105 to 110 degrees.

To counterbalance the enervating effects of heat, try a short cold shower following a hot bath or sauna. Cold water has a tonifying and rejuvenating effect. Cold showers or baths should be around 60 degrees, or as cold as you can tolerate. You might need to add ice cubes to a foot bath or sitz bath to bring it down to the desired temperature.

Combining alternating hot and cold temperatures is the best method for stimulating circulation and lymphatic flow. A simple daily hydrotherapy treatment is to finish your morning shower by standing under a stream of hot water, and then to end with a blast of pure cold water. The key is to get really warm under the hot shower, so that the final cold shower is a welcome treat!

Temperature Ranges for Hydrotherapy Baths

105-110	Very hot (uncomfortable, but tolerable for brief periods)
98-104	Hot (skin turns red)
93-97	Warm (comfortable bath temperature)
81-92	Tepid (just below skin temperature)
66-80	Cool (produces chilly feeling)
55-65	Cold (uncomfortable, but tolerable for brief periods)

Aromatherapy: Fragrance for Purification and Rejuvenation

The healing art of aromatherapy is a perfect complement to the treatments used in hydrotherapy. The fragrant essential oils used in aromatherapy provide a variety of health benefits, and enable you to enhance the effects you desire while increasing the sensory pleasure of your bath. Essential oils stimulate detoxification, improve circulation and lymphatic flow, relieve congestion, and depending on the fragrances you choose, either energize or relax the body and mind.

Fragrant essential oils are distilled from aromatic plants. It takes a lot of plant material to create an essential oil; for example, almost one ton of rose petals are distilled to make a mere ounce of rose essential oil! These concentrated oils have potent effects on both physical and emotional well-being. Think for a moment of how certain fragrances make you feel—the refreshing scent of peppermint, or the soothing and calming perfume of a rose. Aromas evoke powerful memories, and directly influence emotional states through their effects on the central nervous system. On a physical level, the skin absorbs essential oils through the capillaries at the skin's surface, and these aromatic molecules circulate throughout the body via the bloodstream and lymphatic fluid.

There are a few cautions to observe when using essential oils. Never take essential oils internally unless you have the specific guidance of a qualified health practitioner. Because they are extremely concentrated, essential oils should not be applied undiluted to the skin. I have learned from painful experience that even one drop can cause burning and severe irritation. There are exceptions to this rule, but I have encountered a few people who are so sensitive that even the generally soothing lavender acts as a skin irritant. To be safe, always dilute essential oils before using them. You can dilute essential oils with almond, or another vegetable oil to make a massage oil, or by adding the essential oils to a moisturizer or lotion. When using essential oils in the bath, dilute them with a teaspoon of almond oil or witch hazel. Remember that essential oils are highly concentrated, and a little goes a long way. If you have sensitive skin, try a small amount (diluted) on the inside of your elbow overnight and watch for any reaction such as redness or irritation. Some oils, especially citrus oils (except for grapefruit and neroli), can cause photosensitivity to ultraviolet light. If you use citrus oils, avoid going out into the sun for at least 4 hours following application.

Store essential oils in tightly capped dark glass bottles. Rubber-tipped glass drugstore droppers are perfect for dispensing drops of essential oils, but don't leave the droppers in the oil. Many essential oils will cause the rubber to disintegrate into a sticky mess. Bathroom medicine cabinets are generally not the best environment for your precious oils! Keep your essential oils stored in a cool, dark place, away from heat and light. When stored properly, most essential oils will retain their fragrance and potency for several years. Citrus oils are an exception and should be used within one year.

Essential Oil Preparations

Bath: 5-10 drops to a bathtub of water, diluted in oil or witch hazel

Footbath: 5-10 drops, diluted in witch hazel

Massage Oil: 10 drops per ounce of almond oil

Lotion or Moisturizer: 10 drops per ounce of lotion or moisturizer

Sitz bath: 5-10 drops, diluted in witch hazel

Inhalation: 3 drops in a bowl of hot water

Twelve Purifying Essential Oils

Basil: Sweet, spicy scent. Basil is a potent stimulant that increases circulation and eases muscle and joint aches and pains. It alleviates indigestion, and has antiseptic and expectorant properties and helps to treat congestion, coughs, and colds. Basil is excellent for relieving fatigue and nervous tension. *Do not use during pregnancy.*

Cypress: Spicy, balsamlike scent. The diuretic action of cypress helps to relieve water retention and cellulite. It also improves circulation and is helpful for arthritis.

Eucalyptus: Pungent, camphorous scent. Eucalyptus has powerful antimicrobial and decongestant properties and is excellent for treating colds, flus, and respiratory infections.

Fennel: Sweet, earthy scent reminiscent of anise. Fennel has diuretic properties and helps to relieve water retention and cellulite. It also has carminative and laxative properties and alleviates indigestion, gas, and constipation when used in a massage oil on the abdomen. *Do not use during pregnancy.*

Geranium: Herbaceous, roselike scent. Geranium is believed to help balance hormones and has diuretic properties and is used to treat premenstrual syndrome, cellulite, and water retention. It is also relaxing and helps to relieve anxiety and stress.

Ginger: Spicy, warm, woody scent. Ginger stimulates circulation and is helpful for arthritis, sore muscles, and fatigue. When rubbed on the abdomen in a massage oil, it helps to relieve indigestion, gas, and constipation. Ginger has expectorant action, and helps to relieve colds and congestion.

Grapefruit: Sweet, fresh, citrus scent. Grapefruit has diuretic properties, stimulates lymphatic flow, and is excellent for treating cellulite and water retention. The uplifting fragrance helps to relieve fatigue.

Juniper: Sweet, woodsy fragrance. Juniper increases circulation, has diuretic action, and is used to alleviate cellulite, arthritis, and water retention. It also has antiseptic properties and is helpful for treating colds and flus. *Juniper can irritate the kidneys and should not be used by anyone with kidney disease. Do not use during pregnancy.*

Lavender: Sweet, floral, herbaceous fragrance. Lavender is soothing and balancing and can be used for a wide variety of conditions. It is especially helpful for alleviating fatigue, insomnia, stress, headaches, premenstrual syndrome, and sore muscles.

Marjoram: Warm, spicy, sweet, herbaceous scent. Marjoram has antispasmodic and sedative properties and eases sore muscles, stress, headaches, and insomnia. It has mild laxative effects and helps to relieve constipation when used in a massage oil on the abdomen. *Do not use during pregnancy.*

Peppermint: Potent menthol scent. Peppermint has antimicrobial and expectorant properties and helps to alleviate colds and congestion. The stimulating fragrance relieves fatigue and poor circulation and also soothes indigestion. *Peppermint is powerful and can easily burn the skin or mucous membranes. Use only in small amounts.*

Rosemary: Penetrating, herbaceous, slightly camphorous scent. Rosemary is a strong stimulant and is used to treat poor circulation, arthritis, sore muscles, and cellulite. It has antimicrobial properties, and is also effective for treating colds, flus, and congestion. *Do not use during pregnancy.*

Healing Aplications of Essential Oils

Arthritis: basil, cypress, ginger, juniper, marjoram, rosemary
Baths, alternating hot and cold foot and hand baths, massage oil

Cellulite: cypress, fennel, geranium, grapefruit, juniper, rosemary
Baths, massage oil

Colds: basil, eucalyptus, ginger, juniper, peppermint, rosemary
Baths, massage oil, hot foot baths, steam inhalation

Congestion: basil, eucalyptus, ginger, peppermint, rosemary
Baths, massage oil, steam inhalation

Constipation: fennel, ginger, marjoram
Massage oil, sitz bath

Fatigue: basil, lavender, ginger, grapefruit, peppermint, rosemary
Baths, massage oil

Indigestion/Gas: basil, fennel, ginger, lavender, peppermint
Massage oil

PMS: geranium, lavender
Baths, sitz baths, massage oil

Poor Circulation: cypress, ginger, juniper, peppermint, rosemary
Baths, massage oil, alternating hot and cold foot baths

Sore muscles: basil, ginger, lavender, marjoram, rosemary
Baths, massage oil

Stress: basil, geranium, lavender, marjoram
Baths, massage oil

Water retention: cypress, fennel, geranium, grapefruit, juniper
Baths, massage oil

Hydrotherapy Treatments

Epsom Salts Detoxifying Soak

You'll need:

2 cups Epsom salts (available at any pharmacy)

5-10 drops lavender, marjoram, or essential oil of your choice

1 teaspoon distilled witch hazel

A hot Epsom salts bath has powerful detoxifying properties, and is best taken at least 2 hours after eating. In addition to their purifying benefits, Epsom salts are rich in magnesium, which eases sore muscles and induces relaxation. Try an Epsom salts cleansing soak immediately before bedtime for a peaceful night's sleep.

Fill your bathtub with comfortably hot water, adding 2 cups of Epsom salts to the tub while the water is running. Stir the water with your hand to dissolve the salts. For additional detoxifying benefits, dry brush your body to stimulate circulation before entering the tub. Add 5 to 10 drops of essential oils if desired, diluting in 1 teaspoon of witch hazel and adding to the water just before entering the bath. Disperse the essential oils throughout the water with your hand. Soak for 15 to 30 minutes, immersing as much of your body as possible in the water. Add hot water as needed to maintain a comfortably hot temperature.

As you drain the water from the tub, imagine that any toxins and stress that you have been carrying are being released by your body and are swirling down the drain with the bathwater. Rinse your body gently

with tepid water, pat yourself dry with a soft towel, and climb into bed for a relaxing sleep.

Sea and Earth Mineral Bath

You'll need:

2 cups baking soda

1/2 cup Epsom salts

1/2 cup sea salt

5-10 drops lavender, geranium, or essential oil of your choice

1 teaspoon distilled witch hazel

This bath combines minerals from the sea and earth for a concentrated mineral soak. Ojo Caliente, a spa in northern New Mexico, has a delightful natural soda mineral pool. The addition of baking soda to your bathwater replicates this soothing mineral soak, and will leave your skin soft and smooth.

Fill your bathtub with comfortably warm water. Add the Epsom salts, baking soda, and sea salt to the tub while the water is running, stirring the water with your hand to dissolve the minerals. Add 5 to 10 drops of essential oil if desired, diluting first in 1 teaspoon of witch hazel and stirring the mixture into the bathwater with your hand. Relax in the tub for 15 to 30 minutes, immersing as much of your body as possible in the water. Add hot water as needed to maintain the water at a comfortably warm temperature. Rinse with tepid water, gently pat yourself dry with a soft towel, and rest.

Seaweed Bath

You'll need:

2 ounces of kelp, wakame, or dulse (available at natural foods stores)

Mineral-rich seaweed baths are offered at the finest health and beauty spas for their detoxifying and skin-renewing properties. Spas generally add powdered dried seaweeds to soaking tubs. You can powder dry seaweeds in your blender if you desire, but soaking in a tubful of whole sea fronds is a delightful sensory experience. Dried seaweeds expand when added to water, and 2 ounces will fill your tub with floating seaweeds—you'll feel that you're swimming in the ocean!

Fill your bathtub full of comfortably hot water. Add the seaweeds while the tub is filling, allowing them to soak for 10 minutes to expand fully before stepping into the tub. Treat yourself to a dry brush skin mas-

sage while the seaweeds are soaking, and add additional hot water to the tub if necessary. Enter the bath, covering your body with the sea fronds, and soak for 15 to 20 minutes.

Eucalyptus-Seaweed Detoxifying Soak

You'll need:

1 cup Epsom salts

1 cup baking soda

1/2 cup powdered kelp (grind in blender)

5-10 drops eucalyptus essential oil

1 teaspoon distilled witch hazel

optional: ginger tea (if you have a cold or flu)

This powerful cleansing bath combines the detoxifying benefits of Epsom salts and seaweed with the antiseptic and purifying properties of eucalyptus essential oil. Eucalyptus is an excellent remedy for any type of respiratory illness—try this bath the next time you feel that you might be coming down with a cold or flu. Dilute the eucalyptus oil in witch hazel before adding to the bathwater to prevent any possible skin sensitivity to the concentrated essential oil. Add the mixture just before you enter the bath—essential oils are volatile and will dissipate quickly if added while the hot water is running.

To prepare the bath, grind the kelp into a powder in a blender along with one-half cup of sea salt. Fill your bathtub with comfortably hot water. Add the sea salt and kelp mixture along with the Epsom salts while the tub is filling, stirring the salts into the water to help them dissolve. The seaweed will not dissolve in the water. Combine the eucalyptus essential oil with the witch hazel and add to the tub just before entering, dispersing the mixture through the water with your hand.

Enter the tub, and soak for 20 to 30 minutes, adding hot water as needed to keep the water at a comfortable temperature. Visualize toxins and cold or flu viruses being eliminated by your body as you perspire. Allow the water to drain from the tub, rinse gently with tepid water, pat yourself dry with a soft towel, and rest.

Hot Ginger Tea

You'll need:

3-4 teaspoons chopped, fresh ginger root

2 cups water

honey and lemon to taste, if desired

Simmer ginger root in water in a covered pot for 10 minutes. Let sit for an additional 5 minutes, strain, and add honey and lemon to taste if desired. This tea is excellent for relieving the aches and congestion of a cold or flu.

Cellulite Elimination Bath

You'll need:

2 cups Epsom salts

1 cup baking soda

5 drops juniper essential oil

5 drops grapefruit essential oil

1 teaspoon witch hazel

natural bristle body brush or loofah

optional: 1-2 cups parsley tea

The appearance of cellulite is an indication that the organs of detoxification are not working efficiently. Lack of exercise and poor dietary habits—especially fatty foods, sugar, and caffeine—contribute to the formation of cellulite, along with smoking, excessive alcohol intake, stress, and constipation. A cleansing diet and proper exercise are essential components of a cellulite elimination program, but in most cases, must be accompanied by purifying baths, massage, and cleansing herbs. Although cellulite is a stubborn condition, it can be eliminated with a comprehensive detoxification program.

To prepare the cellulite reducing bath, fill the tub with comfortably hot water, adding the Epsom salts and baking soda while the water is running. Vigorously dry brush your entire body before entering the tub, paying particular attention to the areas where cellulite tends to accumulate—the thighs, buttocks, calves, abdomen, and upper arms. Dilute the juniper and grapefruit essential oils in the witch hazel and add to the bathwater just before entering the tub, dispersing the fragrant oils through the bathwater with your hand. Juniper and grapefruit have diuretic and detoxifying benefits, and are specifically recommended for the treatment of cellulite. If desired, sip 1 to 2 cups of parsley tea while in the bath. Parsley has powerful diuretic properties and assists in detoxification.

You can intensify the benefits of this purifying bath by performing self-massage on the areas of your body that are affected by cellulite. To massage areas of soft cellulite, firmly take hold of the fatty tissue, lifting it away from the muscle beneath. Using a twisting and kneading motion, work deeply to bring circulation to these stagnant areas. For areas of firm cellulite that are difficult to lift away from the muscle beneath, make your hands into fists and vigorously rub the area with your knuckles. Cellulite massage may feel slightly painful. Take care to not bruise yourself, but don't be afraid to massage firmly.

While massaging, use the power of your mind to visualize the fatty waste deposits of cellulite breaking up and being flushed out of your body. Imagine your entire body smooth, toned, and healthy. Soak for 20 to 30 minutes, adding hot water as needed to maintain a comfortably hot temperature. This bath is most effective if you make it hot enough to induce gentle perspiration. Rinse with cool water, directing a spray of cold water to any cellulite prone areas to further stimulate circulation. Your skin should be rosy when you leave the bath, indicating increased circulation thoughout your body. For intensive cellulite detoxification, take this purifying bath twice weekly or as often as every other night during a cleansing program.

Parsley Tea

You'll need:

2 cups water

2 tablespoons chopped, fresh parsley leaves

honey and lemon to taste, if desired

Pour boiling water over parsley leaves. Cover, and allow to steep for 15 minutes. Strain, and add honey and lemon if desired.

Body Purifying Scrub

You'll need:

1/2 cup fine sea salt

1 tablespoon almond oil

5 drops grapefruit essential oil

Once a week, treat yourself to this all-over body cleansing scrub. Fine salt crystals exfoliate dry and dead skin cells, and almond oil moisturizes your skin, leaving it silky smooth. Grapefruit essential oil adds purifying properties as well as imparts a delightful uplifting fragrance. This body scrub can be combined with any of the purifying baths, or can be used in the shower as a special morning treat. Use caution when using oil in the tub or shower, as it makes for slippery footing. Use a rubber tub mat to prevent falls.

Combine the sea salt, almond oil, and grapefruit oil in a small wide-mouth plastic container. Mix well. Dampen your body with warm water. Using approximately 1 tablespoonful of the mixture at a time, massage the scrub with a gentle circular motion into your skin, beginning with your calves and working up your thighs, buttocks, and abdomen, avoiding the genital area. Do not rub vigorously, because the salt can irritate your skin if applied harshly. Work up each arm, massaging across your shoulders and back. Use a light touch over the delicate skin of your breasts and neck, and avoid your face. Remove all traces of salt with warm water, and finish with a cool rinse. Pat dry, and enjoy the luxurious satiny feel of your newborn skin.

Caution:

This scrub should not be used by those with sensitive or broken skin, as the salt and grapefruit essential oil can cause irritation.

Skin-Renewing All-Over Body Exfoliant

You'll need:

1/4 cup uncooked rolled oats, ground

1/4 cup raw almonds, ground

1/4 cup corn flour or fine corn meal

1 tablespoon almond oil

5 drops lavender essential oil

5 drops rosemary essential oil

This luxurious body exfoliant removes dull, dry skin and leaves the body silky smooth. It is gentle enough for all skin types, but to be safe, use a light touch if you have sensitive skin and do not apply to broken, burned, or irritated skin.

Grind the rolled oats and almonds separately into a fine meal in a blender or a coffee grinder. Place in a small plastic container, and add the corn flour, almond oil, and lavender and rosemary essential oils.

Dampen your entire body in a warm shower. Beginning with your calves, scoop up approximately 1 tablespoon of the scrub mixture, and gently massage into your skin with a circular motion. Work up each calf and thigh, and massage your abdomen and buttocks. Massage up each arm and across your shoulders and back, and gently massage your chest and neck. Rinse well with warm water, finishing with a cool rinse. This gentle all-over body scrub can be used once a week to keep your skin fresh and radiant.

Caution:
This body scrub is slippery because of the added oil. Use a rubber tub
mat to avoid slipping in the tub or shower.

Invigorating Herbal Detoxifying Soak

You'll need:

3 tablespoons dried nettle

3 tablespoons dried red clover blossoms

2 tablespoons dried peppermint

5 drops peppermint essential oil

5 drops rosemary essential oil

1 teaspoon distilled witch hazel

12-inch square piece of muslin or a cotton handkerchief

Herbs can be used externally as well as internally for purifying the
body. Nettle and red clover blossoms are gentle cleansing herbs, and
peppermint helps to improve circulation and has stimulating properties.
With this treatment, you are essentially making a bathtub full of herbal
tea. Place the dried herbs in the center of the handkerchief or square of
muslin. Gather the corners of the fabric and tie with a piece of ribbon
or cotton twine, making a loop long enough to hang over your tub
faucet. Hang the packet of herbs over the faucet so that the water can
run through the herbs. Fill the tub with comfortably hot water, and then
remove the herbal packet from the faucet and place in the bathwater.

While waiting for the tub to fill, dry brush your body to enhance the
cleansing effects of the bath. Just before entering the tub, add the essen-
tial oils diluted in 1 teaspoon of witch hazel. Disperse throughout the
water with your hand. To intensify the effects of the treatment, sip a cup
of cleansing herbal tea while soaking in the tub.

Soak in the tub for 15 to 20 minutes, adding hot water as needed to
maintain a comfortable temperature. To enhance the energizing and
stimulating effects, finish with a cold shower. This bath is especially nice
for increasing energy at the end of a long day.

Energizing Cleansing Herbal Tea

You'll need:

2 teaspoons nettle

1 teaspoon peppermint

1 teaspoon red clover

2 cups water

honey and lemon to taste, if desired

Place nettle, peppermint, and red clover into a teapot. Add 2 cups of boiling water, cover, and allow to steep for 10 minutes. Strain and add honey and lemon if desired.

Relaxing Herbal Detoxifying Soak

You'll need:

2 tablespoons nettle

2 tablespoons red clover blossoms

2 tablespoons lavender flowers

2 tablespoons linden flowers

10 drops lavender essential oil

12-inch square piece of muslin or cotton handkerchief

Stress increases the production of internal toxins and hinders the body's detoxification processes. Purification, healing and rejuvenation are more easily accomplished when the body and mind are relaxed. Herbs are wonderful allies not only for detoxification, but also for soothing and calming the body, mind, and spirit. This fragrant bath combines the purifying properties of nettle and red clover blossoms with the relaxing properties of lavender and linden blossoms. This is a wonderful bath to come home to after a stressful day. Brew a cup of cleansing herbal tea, light a candle, and listen to your favorite soothing music to help you relax while purifying your body and mind.

Place the dried nettle, red clover, lavender, and linden in the center of the handkerchief or square of muslin. Gather the corners of the fabric and tie with a piece of ribbon or cotton twine, making a loop long enough to hang over the tub faucet. Hang the packet of herbs over the faucet so that the water runs through the herbs, and fill the tub with hot water. Remove the herbal packet and place in the bathwater.

Add 5 drops of lavender essential oil to 2 tablespoons of almond oil, and massage your entire body with deep, slow, relaxing strokes. Just before entering the tub, add 10 drops of lavender essential oil to the water, dispersing the essential oil through the water with your hand. Soak for 15 to 20 minutes, allowing all of the tension to drain out of your body. Rinse off with tepid water and relax.

Purifying and Relaxing Herbal Tea

You'll need:

1 teaspoon nettle

1 teaspoon red clover

2 teaspoons linden flowers

2 cups water

honey and lemon to taste, if desired

Place nettle, red clover, and linden flowers into a teapot. Add 2 cups of boiling water, cover, and let steep for 10 minutes. Strain and add honey and lemon if desired.

Herbal Deep Detoxifying Bath

You'll need:

2 tablespoons dried yarrow flowers

2 tablespoons dried rosemary leaves

2 tablespoons dried crushed juniper berries

2 tablespoons dried ginger root

12-inch square piece of muslin or cotton handkerchief

5 drops juniper essential oil

5 drops rosemary essential oil

1 teaspoon distilled witch hazel

This powerful deep-cleansing herbal bath treatment is good for fending off a cold or flu. Yarrow and ginger have antimicrobial properties and promote sweating and the elimination of toxins through the skin. Juniper and rosemary also have antimicrobial properties, help to open up the bronchial passages, and stimulate circulation as well as help to ease the muscle soreness that often accompanies viral infections.

Place the dried herbs in the center of the handkerchief or square of muslin. Gather the corners of the fabric together and tie into a ball with a piece of ribbon or string, making a loop long enough to hang over the tub faucet. Hang the herbal packet over the faucet so that the water can run through the herbs. Fill the tub with hot water, remove the herbal packet, and place in the bathwater. Steep for 5 minutes, and then add the rosemary and juniper essential oils, diluted in witch hazel. Disperse the essential oils throughout the bathwater with your hand. Soak in the tub for 15 to 20 minutes, rinse off with tepid water, and towel dry.

To further encourage deep internal cleansing, drink a couple of cups of hot yarrow-peppermint-fennel tea while soaking in the bath. Both yarrow and peppermint have diaphoretic and antimicrobial properties and help to eliminate toxins by stimulating perspiration. Fennel seed has expectorant properties and helps the lungs to expel mucus.

Yarrow-Peppermint-Fennel Cleansing Tea

You'll need:

1 teaspoon dried yarrow tops

1 teaspoon dried peppermint

1 teaspoon bruised fennel seeds

2 cups water

honey and lemon to taste, if desired

Place dried yarrow flower tops, dried peppermint, and fennel seeds in a pot. Pour 2 cups of boiling water over the dried herbs, cover, and let steep for 10 minutes. Strain, and add honey and lemon if desired. Drink up to 3 cups daily.

Lymph-Stimulating Footbath

You'll need:

2 deep buckets large enough to hold both of your feet

2 tablespoons powdered ginger

rosemary essential oil

Alternating hot and cold foot baths help to stimulate lymphatic flow and also relieve tired, aching feet and legs. Fill one bucket with water as hot as you can tolerate and stir in the powdered ginger, and fill the other with ice cold water. Use buckets large enough to comfortably hold both of your feet with the water at least covering your ankles. If possible, find buckets deep enough so that the water will reach to the middle of your calves. The higher the water reaches, the more it will assist lymphatic flow.

Dilute 5 to 10 drops of rosemary essential oil in 1 teaspoon of witch hazel, and add to the hot water. Sit in a comfortable chair and immerse both of your feet in the hot water for 3 minutes. Immediately plunge your feet into the cold bucket for 30 seconds. Repeat the cycle 3 times, ending with the cold water soak.

Cleansing Sitz Bath

You'll need:

2 plastic tubs, large enough for you to sit in comfortably

essential oil of your choice (see suggestions that follow)

witch hazel

Sitz baths alleviate congestion in the abdominal organs and help to stimulate circulation and lymphatic flow in the pelvic region. They take a bit of effort, but are one of the most effective treatments for relieving menstrual cramps, constipation, prostatitis, cystitis, and digestive disorders.

You'll need plastic tubs that are large enough to comfortably hold your buttocks. The aim is to focus the hot and cold treatment on the pelvic region, so the water should reach to your navel, leaving your upper body, legs, and feet out of the water. Fill 1 tub with water as hot as you can tolerate. Fill the other with ice cold water. Add 10 drops of essential oil diluted in 1 teaspoon of witch hazel to the hot bath. Choose your essential oils according to the condition that you are treating. Use lavender or geranium for menstrual cramps, fennel or marjoram for constipation, eucalyptus or juniper for prostatitis or cystitis, and ginger or basil for digestive discomfort.

Immerse your hips in the hot tub for 3 minutes, and then immediately shift to the cold bath for 1 minute. Repeat the cycle 3 times, alternating between the hot and cold tubs, and ending with the cold. For best results, use sitz baths 1 to 3 times daily until the condition you are treating is relieved. During a cleansing program, a series of 3 sitz baths on consecutive days can be taken to stimulate cleansing of the abdominal organs.

Purifying Herbal Inhalation

You'll need:

2 tablespoons dried eucalyptus

2 tablespoons dried peppermint

Herbal steam inhalations help to immediately relieve lung and sinus congestion and are excellent for treating colds, flus, coughs, and bronchitis. Bring 1 and 1/2 quarts of water to a boil in a large pot, turn off the heat, and add the eucalyptus and peppermint. Cover the pot and allow to steep for 10 minutes. Place the pot on a table at a comfortable height so that you can sit in front of it. Remove the lid, and make a towel tent over your head and the pot to capture the steam. Breathe in the herbal steam for 10 minutes, lifting the towel to regulate the flow of steam as necessary.

Steam inhalations can be used several times a day when treating a respiratory infection. During a cleansing program, inhalations can be used as desired to help cleanse the lungs and respiratory passages.

Detoxify with Saunas and Steam Baths

You can greatly enhance your cleansing and detoxification program with the addition of saunas or steam baths. As much as 25 percent of all toxins—including pesticides, solvents, drugs, and heavy metals—are eliminated through the skin. By increasing perspiration, saunas step up your body's efforts to get rid of such poisons. Use saunas or steam baths as often as 3 times a week during a cleansing and detoxification program, and once weekly or every other week on a regular basis to maintain optimal health.

Do not use saunas or steams if you are pregnant, or have high blood pressure, cardiovascular disease, or any other serious health condition without first consulting with your health care practitioner.

For best results, the temperature of the sauna or steam should be moderately hot, between approximately 140 and 160 degrees. Steam baths are often within this temperature range, but saunas are frequently hotter. If a sauna is too hot, try opening the door slightly to lower the temperature. A moderately hot temperature makes it possible to stay in the sauna for 15 to 20 minutes at a time, which stimulates a deep level of detoxification.

For the most effective release of toxins, exercise aerobically for 20 to 30 minutes before entering the sauna or steam. A brisk walk is sufficient—anything that will get your circulation and lymph moving and help to start the detoxification process. In addition, massage your entire body with olive oil just before going into the sauna or steam. An oil massage is traditionally used in Ayurvedic purification treatments to help to eliminate toxins that are stored in the fatty tissues. I enjoy adding grapefruit or juniper essential oils to olive oil for additional detoxifying benefits. Both have purifying and diuretic properties and add a wonderful fragrance to the olive oil. Add 10 drops of each (or 20 drops of a single essential oil) to 2 ounces of extra virgin olive oil. Massage your body with long, smooth strokes, and then enter the sauna.

Plan to remain in the sauna or steam for 3 15-minute sessions, or 2 20-minute sessions. Bring plenty of water—at least 1 quart—to keep yourself well hydrated. The more fluids you drink, the more effectively your body can detoxify.

If at any time you feel dizzy or uncomfortable, leave the sauna, rinse off in a cool shower, and rest.

While in the sauna, perform a lymph-draining massage. Beginning with your feet, massage with a gentle circular motion, moving up your calves, around your knees, and up your thighs. Finish with long stroking movements up the entire leg. Massage up your arms and under your armpits in the same way, around your collarbone, chest, neck, shoulders, and under the jaw. This is also a good time to perform an abdominal massage. Work in a clockwise direction, deeply massaging all of the internal organs. Visualize any toxins that are stored in your body being released and excreted through your perspiration.

After 15 minutes, rinse off with tepid water, and then reenter the sauna for another 15-minute session. Complete 2 or 3 sauna sessions, finishing with a cool shower. Relax after your sauna, and be sure to continue drinking plenty of fluids.

Natural Beauty Treatments

A cleansing program is a perfect opportunity to pamper yourself with luxurious bodycare treatments. The finest health spas always include a variety of facials and bodycare therapies as an integral part of a purification and rejuvenation program. You can create the same luxury for yourself at home with the following recipes.

Herbs for Skin Care

Herbs have long been valued not only for their benefits when taken internally, but also for their healing and beautifying properties when used externally. For the following facial and bodycare recipes, choose herbs and essential oils according to your skin type.

Dry Skin
Herbs: Chamomile, comfrey, elder flower, rose
Essential Oils: Chamomile, sandalwood, lavender
Oily Skin
Herbs: Lavender, peppermint, rosemary, yarrow
Essential Oils: Cypress, cedarwood, lavender

Normal Skin
Herbs: Calendula, lavender, chamomile, rose
Essential Oils: Lavender, geranium, rose

Mature Skin
Herbs: Chamomile, comfrey, lavender, rose, rosemary
Essential Oils: Lavender, rosemary, rose

Sensitive Skin
Herbs: Calendula, chamomile, comfrey, rose
Essential Oils: Chamomile, lavender, rose

Herbal Facial Sauna

An herbal facial sauna is the best method for deep cleansing your skin. The warmth of the steam relaxes your pores, and gentle perspiration washes away impurities. Herbal steams also help to hydrate the skin.

Bring 1 1/2 quarts of water to boil in a large pot. Turn off the heat, and add 4 to 6 tablespoons of the herbal mixture appropriate for your skin type, cover the pot, and allow the herbs to steep for 5 minutes. If you have dry skin, add 1 teaspoon of almond oil to the water.

Place the pot on a table, remove the lid, and make a towel tent over your head and the steaming pot. Stay under the towel for 10 to 15 minutes, allowing the herbal steam to open and cleanse your pores. Lift the towel as necessary to regulate the temperature, and take care not to burn yourself with the steam.

Rinse with tepid water and follow with your regular cleansing routine or a facial mask.

Aromatherapy Facial Sauna

This fragrant steam is even simpler than an Herbal Facial Sauna. Close your eyes, breathe deeply, and enjoy the benefits of the essential oils on your skin and psyche.

Pour 1 1/2 quarts of boiling water into a large, heat-proof bowl. Add 3 drops of an essential oil appropriate for your skin type.

Create a towel tent to capture the steam by covering your head and the bowl with a large towel. Lift the towel as necessary to regulate the temperature, and take care to not burn yourself with the steam. Breathe deeply, allowing the steam to gently cleanse your pores for 10 minutes.

Rinse with tepid water, and follow with your regular cleansing routine or a facial mask.

Aromatherapy Facial Compress

This quick and fragrant facial compress is like a mini-sauna. It's a great way to wake up in the morning and can be used as a part of your regular cleansing routine.

Add 2 drops of lavender, geranium, or sandalwood essential oil to a basin of hot water. Soak a small handtowel or washcloth in the scented hot water, wring out the cloth, and gently compress your face and neck with the cloth. Repeat several times, wringing out the cloth each time in the hot water.

Herbal Cleansing Milks

Milk cleansers are much gentler on your skin than soaps. Making your own herbal cleansing milks is simple. To keep them fresh for more than 1 week, freeze the strained herbal milks in ice cube trays, and pop out a cube to thaw as needed.

For Dry to Normal Skin:

2 tablespoons calendula flowers

1 tablespoon chamomile flowers

1 tablespoon rose petals

1 cup whole milk

Combine calendula flowers, chamomile flowers, and rose petals with milk in a pint-size glass jar. Steep overnight in the refrigerator. Strain and rebottle and store in the refrigerator. Use within 1 week.

For Oily to Normal Skin:

1/2 cup yogurt

1/2 cup filtered water

2 tablespoons lavender

1 tablespoon peppermint

Combine yogurt, filtered water, lavender, and peppermint in a pint-size glass jar. Steep overnight in the refrigerator. Strain and rebottle and store in the refrigerator. Use within 1 week.

To use, dampen your face with warm water. Soak a cotton cosmetic pad in the cleansing milk and gently wipe your face. Repeat several times to thoroughly cleanse your skin. Rinse with warm water, spritz with a toner, and follow with a moisturizer for your skin type.

Gentle Cleansing Grains

These cleansing grains gently exfoliate the top layer of dead skin cells, leaving your skin silky smooth. They can be used daily in place of other cleansers, and make an excellent base for facial masks.

For Dry to Normal Skin:

2 cups rolled oats

1/2 cup almonds

2 tablespoons dried rose petals

2 tablespoons dried comfrey leaves

For Oily Skin:

2 cups rolled oats

1/2 cup almonds

1/2 cup cosmetic clay

2 tablespoons dried lavender flowers

1 tablespoon dried peppermint leaves

1 tablespoon dried comfrey leaves

Using a clean coffee grinder, finely grind the oats, almonds, and herbs in separate batches. Mix well, and add cosmetic clay if desired. Store in a covered container.

To use, mix 1 heaping teaspoon of cleansing grains with enough warm water to make a creamy paste. For dry or mature skin, add 1/2 teaspoon of almond oil if desired. Gently massage the mixture into your skin and rinse well with warm water.

Aromatherapy Facial Mask

This simple mask combines the purifying benefits of clay with fragrant essential oils. Clay masks tend to be drying, but can be used on dry skin with the addition of almond oil or honey.

1/2 teaspoon cosmetic clay

2 teaspoons yogurt

1/2 teaspoon honey or jojoba oil, if desired

essential oil appropriate for your skin type

Combine cosmetic clay with yogurt and 2 drops of an essential oil appropriate for your skin type. Add honey or jojoba oil for a moisturizing mask. Smooth onto clean skin. After 15 minutes, remove with a warm, wet washcloth and rinse thoroughly with warm water. Finish with a cool water rinse, spritz with a toner, and apply a moisturizer.

Strawberry Exfoliating Mask

Strawberries, yogurt, and rosemary essential oil all have gentle exfoliating properties. Use this delightfully fragrant mask once a week to keep your skin looking fresh and radiant.

1 medium strawberry

1 teaspoon yogurt

1 teaspoon *Gentle Cleansing Grains*

2 drops rosemary essential oil

Mash 1 medium strawberry and blend with 1 teaspoon of yogurt until smooth. Add 2 drops of rosemary essential oil and 1 teaspoon or more of Gentle Cleansing Grains *(see recipe p. 222) to make a spreadable mask. Apply to clean skin. After 15 minutes, remove with a warm, wet washcloth and rinse thoroughly with warm water. Finish with a cool water rinse, followed by a spritz of toner and moisturizer.*

Avocado Moisturizing Mask

This rich avocado mask can be used weekly as a treat to nourish dry skin. Mix up a large batch and apply it to your arms and legs if they tend to be dry and flaky.

1 tablespoon ripe avocado

1 teaspoon yogurt

1 teaspoon *Gentle Cleansing Grains*

3 drops sandalwood or lavender essential oil

Mash together 1 tablespoon of a soft, ripe avocado with 1 teaspoon of yogurt. Add 3 drops of sandalwood or lavender essential oil and 1 teaspoon or more of Gentle Cleansing Grains *(see recipe on p. 222) to make a thick, spreadable mask. Apply to clean skin. After 15 minutes, remove with a warm, wet washcloth. Rinse thoroughly with warm, then cool water. Follow with toner and moisturizer.*

Honey-Lavender Mask

Honey is a soothing moisturizer for dry, oily, and normal skin. It acts as a humectant, drawing moisture into the skin. Lavender essential oil is balancing for all skin types.

1 tablespoon honey

3 drops lavender essential oil

Combine 1 tablespoon of honey with 3 drops of lavender essential oil. Dampen your face and neck with warm water, or apply an Aromatherapy Facial Compress *(see recipe, p. 221). Smooth on the honey-lavender mixture. Allow the mask to remain on your skin for 15 minutes, and remove with warm water. Follow with toner and moisturizer.*

Herbal Toners

Use herbal toners after washing your face to remove any remaining traces of cleanser and to soothe your skin. Toners are also refreshing when used as a quick skin cleanser after exercise or in hot weather.

For Dry to Normal Skin:

1 cup distilled witch hazel extract

1 teaspoon each: dried chamomile, calendula, comfrey, elder flowers, and rose petals

1 tablespoon vegetable glycerin, if desired

Combine the witch hazel and herbs in a glass jar with a tight-fitting lid. Allow the mixture to steep for 2 weeks in a warm, dark place. Gently shake the jar every day to keep the herbs from settling. Strain, and add 1 tablespoon of vegetable glycerin if desired for extra moisturizing properties. Store in a clean glass bottle. Shake well before using. To use, saturate a cotton ball or pad with toner and apply to skin.

For Oily to Normal Skin:

1 cup distilled witch hazel extract

1 teaspoon each: dried yarrow, peppermint, chamomile, lavender, and comfrey

Combine ingredients in a glass jar with a tight-fitting lid and allow the mixture to steep for 2 weeks in a warm, dark place. Gently shake the jar every day to keep the herbs from settling. Strain, and store in a clean glass bottle. Shake well before using. To use, saturate a cotton ball or pad with the toner and apply to skin.

Aromatherapy Toner

Make a couple of bottles of this toner to keep at home, and for your car, or at work, for a quick spritz of refreshment for your skin and your spirit throughout the day.

1 teaspoon distilled witch hazel

30 drops essential oil appropriate for your skin type

filtered water

In a 6-ounce glass spritzer bottle, combine 1 teaspoon of distilled witch hazel with 30 drops of an essential oil (or combination of essential oils) appropriate for your skin type. Shake vigorously to dissolve the essential oils in the witch hazel, and fill the bottle with filtered water. Shake before using.

Aromatherapy Facial Oil

Pure jojoba oil is an excellent facial moisturizer. Because it is similar to the skin's natural oils, it is easily absorbed. Fragrant essential oils balance and rejuvenate the skin.

1 ounce jojoba oil

10-20 drops essential oil appropriate for your skin type

Combine 10 to 20 drops of an essential oil (or combination of essential oils) appropriate for your skin type with 1 ounce of jojoba oil in a glass bottle. A glass pharmacy bottle with a dropper works well for dispensing droplets of oil. Cleanse your skin, apply a toner, and massage 3 to 4 drops of the moisturizing oil into your damp skin.

Stimulating Scalp Massage

Refresh and cleanse your scalp with this blend of stimulating essential oils. As an extra benefit, rosemary and basil are energizing fragrances and promote mental clarity.

2 drops rosemary essential oil

2 drops basil essential oil

1 teaspoon distilled witch hazel

Combine 2 drops each of rosemary and basil essential oils with 1 teaspoon of distilled witch hazel extract. Massage the mixture into your scalp with your fingers, using gentle, circular movements. Briskly tap your scalp with your fingertips and tug your hair gently at the roots to stimulate circulation.

Scalp-Conditioning Treatment

This conditioning treatment helps to maintain a healthy scalp and promotes hair growth. Apply approximately 30 minutes before shampooing.

2 ounces jojoba oil

20 drops rosemary essential oil

10 drops lavender essential oil

In a glass bottle, combine jojoba oil with rosemary and lavender essential oils. Shake well. To use, apply 1/2 teaspoon or more to your scalp, massaging in with your fingertips. Leave on for 30 minutes or even overnight, if desired. Shampoo and condition as usual.

Deep-Conditioning Hair Treatment

A deep conditioning treatment helps to restore softness and shine to dull, dry hair.

2 ounces olive oil

2 ounces jojoba oil

20 drops rosemary essential oil

1-2 teaspoons honey

Pour the olive and jojoba oils into a glass bottle. Add the rosemary essential oil and shake well.

Dampen your hair with warm water. Gently heat 1 to 2 teaspoons of honey and 1 to 2 tablespoons of the oil mixture to a comfortably warm temperature. Massage the warm oil mixture into your scalp with your fingertips. Work the oil through your hair all the way to the ends.

Cover your hair with a shower cap and a hot, damp towel to help the oils penetrate the hair. Leave in place for 30 minutes, replacing the hot towel as it cools.

Shampoo twice to remove the conditioning treatment, and follow with a small amount of your usual conditioner if necessary.

Herbal Hair Rinse

Use this herbal rinse after shampooing and conditioning to freshen your scalp and give body to your hair.

Normal hair (dark): Rosemary, sage, lavender

Normal hair (light): Chamomile, calendula

Dry hair: Chamomile, comfrey

Oily hair: Nettle, yarrow, thyme, sage

Dandruff: Sage, thyme, nettle, lavender

Choose any combination of the above herbs. Bring 1 quart of water and 4 tablespoons of the dried herbal mixture to a boil over medium heat in a covered pot. Turn off the heat and allow to steep until cool.

Strain out the herbs and use 1/2 cup as a final rinse after shampooing and conditioning. For extra fragrance, add 3 drops of lavender essential oil to the hair rinse before applying it to your hair.

If you have dry hair, mix the herbal rinse with a conditioner and apply, then rinse out. Store remaining herbal rinse in the refrigerator for up to 1 week.

Softening Foot Soak

Treat your feet to a little pampering with this softening and fragrant foot soak.

1/2 cup baking soda

1/2 cup borax

5 drops lavender essential oil

rose petals

Fill a plastic tub large enough to comfortably hold your feet with hot water. Stir in 1/2 cup of baking soda and 1/2 cup of borax, both of which are natural skin softeners and fresheners. Add 5 drops of lavender essential oil and a handful of rose petals if you have them.

Soak your feet for 10 minutes to soften calluses. While your feet are still damp, gently remove calluses with a pumice stone or callus file. Clean under your toenails, and push back your cuticles with an orangewood stick. Pat your feet dry, and trim your toenails. File gently to smooth rough nail edges, and apply Nail Nourishing Oil *(see recipe that follows).*

Aromatherapy Nail Soak

A warm herbal soak with fragrant essential oils softens your hands and makes it easy to shape up your nails and cuticles.

1 tablespoon calendula flowers

1 tablespoon chamomile flowers

1 teaspoon almond oil

5 drops lavender essential oil

Make an herbal infusion by pouring 2 cups of boiling water over calendula and chamomile flowers. Allow to steep until comfortably warm and strain into a bowl. Add almond oil and lavender essential oil.

Soak your hands in the warm bath for 10 minutes. Clean under your nails, and push back your cuticles with an orange wood stick while your hands are damp.

Pat your hands dry, and trim and file your nails. Massage Nail Nourishing Oil *(see recipe that follows)* into your nails and cuticles, and buff your nails with a natural chamois buffer.

Nail Nourishing Oil

Nails become brittle and dry when exposed to hot water, soaps, and nail polishes or other chemicals. Massage a few drops of this protective oil into your nails and cuticles in the morning and evening.

2 tablespoons jojoba oil

2 tablespoons almond oil

15 drops sandalwood essential oil

Combine jojoba oil with almond oil in a 1-ounce glass bottle with a dropper. Add sandalwood essential oil. Shake well to blend.

Massage 3 to 4 drops into nails and cuticles. Buff with a chamois buffer if desired to heighten the natural shine of your nails.

Aromatherapy Body Oil

Smooth a few drops of this massage oil over your entire body immediately after emerging from a shower or bath while your skin is still damp. The oil seals moisture into your skin and creates a protective barrier against dryness.

4 ounces almond oil

2 ounces jojoba oil

50 drops (1/2 teaspoon) essential oil of your choice

Combine the almond and jojoba oils in a glass bottle and add 1/2 teaspoon of the essential oil of your choice. Use one essential oil, or combine 2 or 3 for a total of 1/2 teaspoon. Shake well.

Use as a massage oil, or as a moisturizer after bathing.

Essential Oils for Massage: chamomile, clary sage, geranium, grapefruit, jasmine, lavender, neroli, patchouli, rose, sandalwood, ylang ylang

Silken Body Powder

Body dusting powders add an elegant finishing touch to a bath. They give your skin a silky feel, and absorb excess perspiration.

1 cup arrowroot powder

1/2 cup white cosmetic clay

1/2 cup rose petals or lavender flowers

sandalwood, rose, or lavender essential oil

Powder the rose petals or lavender flowers in a clean coffee grinder. Mix the arrowroot, clay, and powdered roses or lavender together.

Add approximately 50 drops of essential oil, and thoroughly mix the oil into the powder with your fingertips. Store in a covered tin or glass jar, and allow the powder to mellow for several days before using.

Apply with a powder puff or soft brush, or package in spice jars with shaker tops.

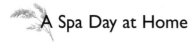

A Spa Day at Home

Make time in your life each week to create your own at-home spa experience. Set aside at least 2 hours if you can, but even if you have only 1 hour, you can indulge in a variety of bodycare treatments that will refresh and renew your body, mind, and spirit.

Gather together everything you will need; your skin, hair, and bodycare products and a thick bathtowel and robe are essentials. Some nice extras include a bath pillow, candles, incense, and soothing music. Brew a cup of your favorite herbal tea or make a glass of fresh fruit or vegetable juice, turn off the phone, and put a "Do Not Disturb" sign on the door. You deserve this uninterrupted time to nurture your body and spirit.

1. Begin with a *Stimulating Scalp Massage* or a *Deep Conditioning Hair Treatment.*

    Time required: 5 minutes

2. Wash your face with an *Herbal Cleansing Milk* or gentle cleanser of your choice and warm water.

    Time required: 2 minutes

3. Deep cleanse your skin with an *Herbal* or *Aromatherapy Facial Sauna.* If time is limited, use an *Aromatherapy Facial Compress.*

    Time required: 10 minutes (2 minutes for *Facial Compress*)

4. Apply a *Strawberry Exfoliating Mask* to your face and neck. With the mask in place, treat your feet to a *Softening Foot Soak.* Clean and trim your toenails and cuticles and pumice away rough spots on your heels.

    Time required: 15 minutes

5. Remove the *Strawberry Exfoliating Mask* with a warm, wet washcloth. Apply an *Avocado Moisturizing Mask* or a *Honey-Lavender Mask.*

   Time required: 5 minutes

6. Fill the bathtub with warm water. While you're waiting for the tub to fill, briskly dry brush the skin over your entire body with a natural bristle body brush.

   Time required: 5 minutes

7. Choose a bath treatment from the Hydrotherapy recipes, or simply add 10 drops of lavender essential oil to the bathwater. Add 1 cup of baking soda to soften the water if desired, and 1 teaspoon of almond oil if your skin tends to be dry. Soak, relax, and enjoy. Visualize any tension flowing out of your body and mind.

   Time required: 15 minutes

8. If desired, apply an all-over exfoliating body scrub from the Hydrotherapy recipes to polish and smooth your body. Remove the moisturizing mask from your face with a warm, wet washcloth. Shampoo and condition your hair, and follow with an *Herbal Hair Rinse* if desired. Shower off using warm water, and finish with an invigorating cool rinse.

   Time required: 15 minutes

9. Pat your skin dry and apply an *Aromatherapy Massage Oil* or moisturizer while your skin is still damp. Spritz your face with an *Aromatherapy Toner* and apply an *Aromatherapy Facial Oil.*

   Time required: 5 minutes

10. Soak your hands in an *Aromatherapy Nail Soak* and clean and push back your cuticles with an orange stick. Trim and file your nails, apply *Nail Nourishing Oil,* and buff to a gloss.

    Time required: 10 minutes

chapter sixteen

How to Use Breathing, Massage and Rest to Eliminate Toxins

Purify Your Body with Your Breath

Breathing is one of the most important aspects of a cleansing and rejuvenation program. Deep breathing brings healing oxygen to every cell of the body, while eliminating gaseous metabolic wastes. Rhythmical deep breathing also directly affects the nervous system, engendering a relaxation response that has a positive effect on the entire body. Although breathing is primarily an involuntary process, it is largely within our conscious control. The breath links the mind and body, and when you focus your attention on your breath, you immediately and positively affect your physical and emotional well-being.

During times of emotional or physical stress, the automatic response is to breathe shallowly. This causes a build-up of carbon dioxide and other toxins in the body, and limits the amount of oxygen that the cells are receiving. Many people get into the habit of breathing shallowly all the time and rarely take a full, deep breath. The lungs begin to lose their elasticity, toxins build up in the bloodstream, tissues, and cells, and physical and emotional health deteriorate.

Learning to breathe fully is one of the quickest ways to energize and heal your body and relax your mind. Try the following 1-minute exercise to experience the immediate benefits of deep breathing: Focus your attention on your breath, and inhale as you normally do through your nose. Open your mouth slightly, and make your exhalation a bit longer than your inhalation. Again, inhale through your nose, and exhale through your slightly open mouth, consciously extending your exhalation. Practice this for a few minutes, and then return to normal breathing. This simple exercise empties the lungs and helps to clear the bloodstream of carbon dioxide, slows down your rate of breathing to bring about a feeling of relaxation, and automatically increases the amount of oxygen that you inhale.

Take time every day to practice at least a few minutes of breathing exercises. Try the exercises in this chapter, and choose your favorites. Once you become familiar with conscious breathing techniques, you can practice them anywhere, at any time. I use a variety of breathing exercises, from early morning cleansing breaths to the deep, diaphragmatic breathing that I practice at night while lying in bed. Throughout the day, I often bring my awareness to my breathing, and spend a minute or two consciously using my breath to energize, heal, and relax my body.

If you've never practiced deep-breathing exercises before, you might find that you feel a bit lightheaded at the beginning. Go slowly with the exercises and work at a pace that is comfortable for you.

Diaphragmatic Breathing

Most people get into the habit of breathing shallowly, which fills only the top portion of the lungs. After years of breathing in this constricted way, the lungs begin to lose their elasticity. Deep diaphragmatic breathing, also called abdominal or belly breathing, encourages breathing into the lower portion of the lungs and fully oxygenates the body. Watch a young child breathe, and you'll get the idea of how you should be breathing. When you inhale, your abdomen should expand, and when you exhale, your abdomen should contract. This is just the opposite of how most adults breathe; chronic stress and internalizing messages such as "hold in your stomach" lead to poor breathing habits. To restore a healthy breathing pattern, practice the following exercise.

Lie comfortably on your back. Relax for a moment, consciously letting go of any tension. Place a book over your navel to help to focus your attention on your abdomen. Inhale, and push your abdomen up toward the ceiling. As you exhale, pull your abdominal muscles in toward your spine. You should feel the book rising and falling with your breath. Repeat this 3 times, and then relax. On the next inhalation, allow your abdomen to expand, but without pushing. Exhale, and allow your abdomen to gently and naturally contract. Repeat 3 times, again observing the book rising and falling with your breath.

Remove the book, and inhale to a long, slow, comfortable count of 6, allowing your abdomen to expand, and exhale slowly to a count of 6, allowing your abdomen to contract. Continue to breathe in this way for a few minutes, and then relax.

Complete Breath

The complete breath fills the lower, middle, and upper portions of the lungs with oxygen. This exercise increases lung capacity, helps to restore elasticity to the lungs, and cleanses the blood.

Lie comfortably on your back. Breathe slowly and rhythmically, concentrating on inhaling and exhaling a continuous stream of air. Begin inhaling slowly, and fill the lower part of your lungs, gently expanding your abdomen. As you continue to inhale, expand your stomach area and lower chest to bring your breath up into the middle portion of your lungs. Continue to inhale, and bring your breath into the upper portion of your lungs by expanding your upper chest and ribs. Hold the complete breath for a moment, and then gently and slowly exhale in the reverse order, allowing the air to flow out of the upper, middle and lower lungs. Slightly contract your abdomen at the end of the breath to completely clear your lungs. Pause for just a moment, and then begin the cycle again. Make your breath steady and rhythmic, imagining your breath flowing into your lungs like a warm ocean wave, and then flowing out. Continue breathing in this deep, rhythmical manner for a couple of minutes, until your body is deeply relaxed.

Recharge Breath

This quick breathing exercise can be practiced anywhere to relieve tension and to help restore a healthy breathing pattern. Sit comfortably on the floor or in a chair with your spine straight. Inhale deeply, filling your lungs as fully as possible while relaxing your abdominal muscles to allow your abdomen to expand. Open your mouth slightly, and exhale, blowing all of the air out of your lungs until every bit of air has been exhaled. At the same time, draw your abdomen in sharply to help press out the air. Repeat between 3 to five times.

Vitality-Enhancing Breath

This simple energizing breath cleanses your lungs of stale air and provides a burst of renewed vitality. Sit or stand with your spine straight and your shoulders relaxed. Inhale a series of short, quick breaths through the nostrils until your lungs are completely filled. Exhale forcefully and quickly through your mouth, making the sound "ha" as you exhale completely. Repeat several times, and then resume normal breathing.

Deep-Cleansing Breath

This powerful breathing exercise helps to cleanse the lungs and bloodstream. Sit cross-legged on the floor with your spine straight and your shoulders relaxed. Inhale and exhale deeply a few times through the nose to relax your body and mind and to establish a comfortable breathing rhythm. As you inhale, gently expand your abdomen, and as you exhale, gently contract your abdomen.

Now exhale deeply and forcefully through your nose, at the same time pulling your abdominal muscles sharply in toward your spine. The chest, shoulders, neck, and face remain relaxed. Focus on expelling as much stale air from your lungs as possible during the exhalation. Your lungs will naturally fill following this powerful exhalation.

Repeat several times, increasing to 10 or 15 repetitions as you are comfortable. After the last exhalation, take a slow, deep inhalation, exhale slowly, and relax.

Alternate Nostril Breathing

This calming breathing exercise cleanses the respiratory tract, relaxes the nervous system, and promotes clarity of thought. Sit in a comfortable position with your spine straight and your shoulders relaxed.

Gently press your right nostril closed with your right thumb and inhale slowly and deeply through your left nostril. Gently press your left nostril closed with the ring finger of your right hand. Retain the breath for a few seconds, and then release your thumb, exhaling slowly and completely through the right nostril. Immediately inhale through the right nostril with a slow and steady rhythm. Close your right nostril with your right thumb and retain the breath for a few seconds. Release your ring finger, and exhale slowly and steadily through your left nostril. Repeat at least 10 times, always keeping your breath even and controlled.

Abdominal Cleansing Breath

This advanced breathing technique is used in yoga to increase energy in the abdomen, massage the digestive organs, and stimulate the release of toxins from the intestinal tract. Practice this exercise on an empty stomach.

Stand in a comfortable position with your feet about a foot apart. Take a deep inhalation, and bend slightly forward from your waist, placing your hands on your lower thighs. Exhale completely through your mouth, releasing all of the air from your lungs. Press your palms firmly against your thighs, and sharply draw your abdomen upward and back toward your spine. Without taking a breath, allow your abdomen to relax, and then immediately draw it in again. Repeat this pumping action 10 to 20 times. Rest for a moment, allowing your breathing to return to normal. Repeat the entire sequence 5 to 10 times.

The Rejuvenating Benefits of Massage

If massage is not already a regular part of your life, a cleansing program is a perfect opportunity to treat yourself to the rejuvenating benefits of this ancient healing art. Massage is one of the great pleasures in life—and it's good for you, as well! Massage relaxes tight muscles, stimulates the flow of both blood and lymph, enhances the elimination of toxins from tissues, and calms the nervous system. On the surface of the body, massage helps to sweep away dead skin cells, promoting a healthy glow.

Simple massage techniques such as a dry brush massage or a hot towel scrub can easily become a part of your daily routine. Either 1 takes less than 5 minutes, and will greatly improve your skin texture and enhance the flow of blood and lymph. For deep, rejuvenative, and detoxifying benefits, give yourself the gift of a full body massage once a week or every other week on a regular basis. Find a massage therapist you enjoy working with, or exchange massages with your partner or a friend. For suggestions for books and videotapes on massage, see the Resource section.

Dry Brush Massage

This quick massage technique takes only a few minutes and is an excellent daily routine for stimulating lymphatic flow and surface circulation. Skin brushing also removes the buildup of dead cells on the surface of the skin and improves skin texture and appearance. When performed daily, skin brushing helps to eliminate cellulite.

You'll need a soft vegetable bristle brush that is stiff enough to stimulate your skin, but not so rough that it causes irritation. Find a brush that feels just right to you. A brush with a long detachable handle is nice to have so that you can easily reach your back.

A good time to perform a dry brush massage is just before showering or bathing. Brush vigorously, but not so hard that you scratch your skin. Begin with a light touch, and increase the pressure as you become accustomed to the massage. To stimulate lymphatic flow, brush with long sweeping strokes, moving in the direction of your heart. Avoid sensitive areas such as the genitals, nipples, and face, and avoid any areas where the skin is irritated. Begin with the soles of your feet, and brush up your calves, behind your knees, up your thighs, and over your hips to your lower back. Brush your hands, up the front and backs of your arms, across your shoulders, down your chest, gently over your breasts, and down the back of your neck and upper back. Finish by brushing your abdomen with a clockwise circular motion.

Hot Towel Scrub

A hot towel scrub is an excellent early morning ritual, or is just as appropriate to use before going to sleep. This massage technique cleanses the skin, enhances circulation, and improves lymphatic flow.

You'll need a rough cotton terry washcloth and a basin of very hot water. Add 3 drops of lavender essential oil and mix into the water with your hand. Dip the washcloth in the hot water, and wring it out. Beginning with your feet, rub the soles, between your toes, and over the tops of your feet. Rub briskly to stimulate circulation—you should immediately see a healthy, rosy glow. Work up your calves, behind your knees, and up your thighs in the direction of your heart. Wring the washcloth out in the water frequently to keep the cloth hot. Massage your hands, up your arms, across your shoulders, down your chest and around your breasts. Rub down your neck and back, and finish by rubbing in a clockwise circular motion over your abdominal area.

This scrub can also be performed with cold water as a wonderful morning wake-up and toner.

Lymph-Cleansing Massage

Lymph bathes and purifies all of the tissues of the body and is responsible for carrying toxins out of the cells. The intricate network of lymph glands located throughout the body filters toxins from the lymph and is an integral part of the immune system. Because the lymphatic system has no pump, it relies on external help—such as exercise or massage—to help move it through the lymphatic channels. Lymph stagnation is common, and results in fatigue, cellulite, and increased susceptibility to infections. Massage is excellent for stimulating lymphatic flow because the lymph flows just beneath the surface of the skin. The release of toxins is greatly accelerated by massage, so be sure to drink plenty of water or a cleansing herbal tea after a treatment.

I like to use a purifying massage oil to enhance the benefits of a lymphatic massage. Add 20 drops of a detoxifying essential oil such as grapefruit, juniper, cypress, or fennel to two ounces of almond or olive oil. Long, sweeping massage strokes in the direction of the heart will help to move the lymph through the lymphatic channels. Use small, gentle, circular movements in areas where lymph nodes are concentrated, such as behind the knees, in the groin and abdominal area, under the armpits, around the collarbone, and in the neck.

Working on one leg at a time, begin by massaging your foot with your fingertips, using gentle, circular movements. Visualize every cell of your body being bathed and purified by the lymph. With long, sweeping movements, stroke up your foot and calf, drawing the flow of lymph upward. Work with gentle circular movements behind your knee, and then draw the lymph up toward your groin by stroking up your thigh. Perform the same massage on your other leg. When you reach the groin, work on both sides of the groin at the same time, using gentle circular movements to thoroughly massage and cleanse the many lymph nodes in this area. With sweeping strokes, bring the lymph up toward your abdomen, and massage your abdominal area with a gentle, smooth clockwise motion.

Move to your neck, and using your fingertips, massage in a circular motion around the back of your neck at the base of your skull, under your jaw, and down the sides of your neck. Make gentle stroking movements down your neck to your collarbone, and massage with circular movements all around your collarbone and down the center of your chest. Finish with feathery, sweeping strokes in this area.

Working on one arm at a time, begin by massaging your hand and fingers, and draw the flow of lymph up toward your elbow with gentle strokes along your inner and outer arm. Massage around the inside of your elbow, and stroke the lymph up toward your underarm, massaging the lymph nodes in the armpit with a gentle, circular motion. Draw the lymph out from under the arm with a stroking motion, moving over the breast and toward the center of your chest. Massage under the breasts, again drawing the lymph to the center of your chest. Visualize the lymphatic channels being cleansed and purified, and all toxins being released from your cells as you perform this cleansing massage.

Cellulite Massage

Cellulite is a common condition that appears as lumpy fat on the thighs, buttocks, abdomen, and upper arms. While exercise and a cleansing diet are essential for eliminating cellulite, massage will greatly speed the process. Cellulite is an indication of stagnant lymphatic flow and impaired detoxification. The deep, strong strokes of cellulite massage help to release the accumulation of waste materials that manifest as cellulite. For best results, perform cellulite massage daily, or even twice daily.

Begin your cellulite massage with a few minutes of dry brush massage to stimulate lymphatic flow. Apply a purifying massage oil made by adding 20 drops of a detoxifying essential oil such as grapefruit, fennel, juniper, or cypress to 2 ounces of olive or almond oil. The essential oils will penetrate the fatty tissues and help to eliminate the toxins that contribute to cellulite.

Apply the purifying oil with smooth, gliding strokes onto the area that you will be massaging. Always stroke in the direction of your heart to enhance proper lymphatic flow and blood circulation. To massage areas of soft cellulite, firmly grasp the fatty tissue, lifting it away from the muscle beneath. Using a twisting and kneading motion, work deeply, squeezing the tissue to help break down the fatty deposits. Don't bruise yourself, but work as deeply as you can. For areas of firm cellulite that are difficult to separate from the muscle beneath, make your hands into fists and briskly rub the area with your knuckles. Cellulite massage may feel slightly painful, but needs to be vigorous to be effective. The area that you are working on should turn rosy with increased circulation. This indicates that blood and lymph are flowing into the tissues, cleansing toxins from the cells and carrying away waste deposits.

While massaging, use the power of your mind to visualize the fatty waste deposits breaking up and being flushed out of your body. See your body as smooth, firm, and toned. Finish your massage with long, firm, smooth strokes in the direction of your heart.

Abdominal Massage

An abdominal massage enhances the elimination of toxins by stimulating the function of the digestive organs and the large intestine. This massage should be performed on an empty stomach—first thing in the morning is ideal. Lie comfortably on your back, with your knees bent to relax your abdominal area. Apply massage oil to your abdomen. To make a massage oil that will stimulate intestinal function, add 10 drops of fennel, marjoram, or ginger essential oil to 1 ounce of olive or almond oil.

Begin by massaging your liver and spleen, which are located just beneath your ribs. Massage as deeply as you comfortably can with smooth, gliding strokes in the direction of your intestines. Tenderness in this area or any other organ indicates unreleased energy and the accumulation of toxins. Continue to gently massage the area, breathing into the tension and visualizing the area filled with white, purifying, healing light. Move to your stomach, and use your fingers and the palms of your hands to make slow, downward strokes.

Place your left hand on top of your right, and with a firm, circular motion, begin massaging at the right lower side of your abdomen. Massage as deeply as you comfortably can, again paying attention to any tender spots and using your breath and the power of visualization to dissolve any accumulation of tension and toxins. Move in small increments up the right side of your abdomen, across your belly just above the navel, down the left side of your abdomen, and across your pelvis. Finish by massaging your abdomen with smooth, gliding strokes in a clockwise direction to stimulate large intestine function. Rub your hands together briskly to stimulate energy flow, and place your palms over your abdominal area, imagining your entire abdomen filled with healing light.

Aromatherapy Massage Oils

It's simple to create your own custom blends of aromatherapy massage oils. Essential oils not only add a delightful fragrance to a massage blend, but they also impart healing properties which are absorbed through the skin and into the tissues. See p. 205 in Chapter 15 for more specific information on essential oils.

Stimulating Oils: Basil, ginger, rosemary

Detoxifying Oils: Cypress, fennel, grapefruit, juniper

Relaxing Oils: Lavender, geranium, sandalwood, clary sage, rose, jasmine, ylang ylang, chamomile

To make a massage oil, add 10 drops of essential oil to 1 ounce of vegetable oil. My favorite oils to use for massage are extra virgin olive oil or expeller-pressed almond oil. Extra virgin olive oil is very stable and does not need to be refrigerated, but has a definite olive scent. I generally use olive oil for massage before a sauna or a bath. Almond oil has a light scent and is also excellent as a massage oil, but needs to be refrigerated. Other more expensive but good choices for massage oils include apricot, hazelnut, jojoba, and sesame seed oils. Jojoba oil is actually a liquid wax, and like olive oil, is resistant to oxidation and rancidity. You can add approximately 10 percent of jojoba oil to any other massage oil blend to help to prevent rancidity.

Try the following massage oil blends, and have fun creating your own!

Lymph-Purifying Massage Oil
4 ounces extra virgin olive oil or expeller pressed almond oil
15 drops cypress essential oil
15 drops juniper essential oil
10 drops lemon essential oil

Anticellulite Massage Oil
4 ounces extra virgin olive oil or expeller pressed almond oil
20 drops juniper essential oil
20 drops grapefruit essential oil

Massage Oil for Constipation
4 ounces extra virgin olive oil
30 drops marjoram essential oil
10 drops ginger essential oil

Relaxing Massage Oil
4 ounces expeller pressed almond or apricot oil
20 drops lavender essential oil
20 drops sandalwood essential oil

Massage Oil for Sore Muscles
4 ounces extra virgin olive oil or expeller pressed almond oil
20 drops rosemary essential oil
20 drops basil essential oil

The Restorative Benefits of Rest

Rest = Restoration. It makes sense, doesn't it? While exercise and movement are essential for stimulating circulation and the elimination of toxins, rest and sleep provide an opportunity for the body to cleanse, repair, and rejuvenate on a deep cellular level. Most people in our society are chronically sleep deprived. Use your detoxification program as an opportunity to nourish your body with plenty of healing sleep and rest.

Napping for More Energy

Many people allow themselves the luxury of a nap only if they are sick. But the body has natural cycles of rest and activity, and the desire for a few minutes of rest in the midafternoon seems to be an inherent physiological need. Although most people in our culture fight the desire for rest and even view it as a sign of indolence, in many cultures, a midday siesta is regarded as a necessity.

Taking a few minutes out of the day for a nap can be wonderfully restorative. When you stop all activity to close your eyes and rest, both your body and your mind have an opportunity to relax deeply. Taking naps during a detoxification program is especially helpful for maintaining a state of calm and rest that facilitates deep cleansing.

The best time to nap is usually in the mid-afternoon, approximately 8 hours after you arise and 8 hours before you go to bed at night. For most people, this coincides with the time that they naturally feel the desire to nap—somewhere around 3:00 P.M. If you nap too late in the afternoon, you may have difficulty going to sleep at night. Try to cultivate the habit of napping at the same time each day, and for the same length of time. This helps to get your body into a comfortable napping rhythm. When you nap, make yourself as comfortable as possible. Take off your shoes, loosen tight items of clothing, find a comfortable chair or couch, and dim the lights in the room. Even if you don't sleep, take a few minutes to treat your body and your mind to a deep relaxation exercise. For example, focus on your breathing and progressively relax every muscle in your body, beginning with your toes and moving slowly up through your body to your scalp. See Chapter 17 for more suggestions for relaxation exercises. For most people, naps of between 15 to 30 minutes are the most refreshing. Upon awakening, take a minute or two to stretch, walk around, and spritz your face with cool water or an aromatherapy toner to help to relieve any feelings of momentary grogginess.

The Healing Power of Sleep

Much of the body's healing work takes place while you sleep. Without the need to attend to all of the functions of daily life, your immune system and organs of detoxification can focus attention on cleansing and restoration. This is the time when your body does major housecleaning, taking care of wastes that have accumulated during the day and repairing cellular damage. Cultivate the habit of going to bed early, before 10 P.M. When dark falls, the body naturally wants to sleep. Overriding this desire for sleep interferes with the natural rhythm of cleansing. According to traditional Chinese and Ayurvedic medicine, as well as Western naturopathic healing philosophy, the most important hours for detoxification and rejuvenation are before midnight. The earlier you go to bed, the better.

For the most restful and restorative sleep, make sure that your sleeping environment is as healthful as possible. Use natural cotton bedding to allow your body to breathe, and wear comfortable, loose cotton sleepwear if you wear anything at all. Keep your window open at least a few inches year round to provide plenty of fresh air. Avoid eating for at least two hours before sleeping. This ensures that your body's energy can be used for healing and rejuvenation instead of for digestion. If you do want to eat something before bed, a piece of fruit is a good choice. Fruit is cleansing and is quickly digested.

If you have difficulty getting to sleep, there are a number of factors to consider that can help you to get a good night's rest. First of all, make sure that you are getting sufficient exercise during the day. A 30-minute walk either before or after dinner is especially helpful for ensuring deep sleep. Avoid caffeine in all forms. While caffeine late in the evening is particulary disruptive for sleep, even a morning cup of coffee can cause nighttime sleep disturbances for some people. Avoid stressful mental activity in the hours right before bed, and spend time relaxing with a good book, enjoyable conversation, or soothing music instead. Make sure that your sleeping environment is peaceful and quiet. If you can't escape noisy neighbors or traffic sounds, invest in a sound machine that creates soothing background "white noise" that masks disturbing sounds.

Natural remedies for restful sleep include soothing baths and herbal teas. Try a warm bath just before bed with 2 cups of Epsom salts and 10 drops of lavender essential oil diluted in the bathwater. Epsom salts are rich in magnesium, which helps to relax the muscles and the nervous system, and lavender has soothing effects on both the body and the mind. A cup of chamomile or passionflower tea also promotes relaxation. Brew a strong tea by pouring 1 cup of boiling water over 2 teaspoons of dried herb and steeping in a covered pot for 15 minutes. Strain, and add honey or lemon if desired. For serious insomnia, try taking 1 teaspoon of valerian or 1/2 teaspoon of kava tincture diluted in a small amount of warm water (or 2 capsules of dried herb) approximately 30 minutes before bed.

Practicing calming breathing and deep relaxation exercises can also help to promote restful sleep by quieting the body and mind. Cultivate the habit of taking a few minutes to purify your body and your mind with your breath when you first get into bed. Simply focus on your breathing, taking 3 deep, relaxing cleansing breaths, and then mentally scan your body for any areas of tension. When you find a pocket of tension, gently breathe into that area, imagining the tension leaving your body with your exhalation. You'll most likely fall asleep in the middle of this deeply relaxing exercise, which is just fine!

Waking up in a pleasant way is just as important as getting a good night's sleep. Leave your shades or curtains open so that the early morning light will signal your body that it's time to rise. If you're going to bed at the same time each night, you'll find that you'll naturally awaken at a regular time each morning. If you do need the help of an alarm, make it a gentle introduction to the day with pleasant music or a soothing chime. Don't leap out of bed, but take a few minutes to stretch and breathe, appreciating the blessing of another day of beautiful life and opportunities that await you.

chapter seventeen

Support Cleansing with the Power of Your Mind

Your mind is a wonderful ally in your cleansing program. Although you cannot see your thoughts, they have powerful effects on your health and well-being. Think of your thoughts as mental nourishment. Just as you choose with care the foods that you eat, begin to choose your thoughts with the same care. Realize that your thoughts do not choose you—you choose your thoughts. The first step in cultivating healthier thinking patterns is to become aware of the habitual thought patterns that you have. We all have mental tapes that run continuously through the subconcious mind. By becoming aware of your habitual thoughts, you can begin to replace the negative, self-defeating thoughts that you have with more positive, life-affirming thoughts. Journal writing, relaxation exercises, and meditation and visualization are powerful techniques for quieting the mind and cultivating healthier ways of thinking.

Journal Writing for Emotional Detoxification

Many times, people know that they are anxious, depressed, or unhappy, but are unable to identify the cause of their unhappiness or are uncertain of how to make changes that will result in a more satisfying life. Unexpressed or unacknowledged feelings are almost always at the root of painful emotional blocks. Journal writing is a simple, and yet extremely powerful tool for emotional detoxification and for cultivating self-understanding.

Even if you are not feeling emotionally stuck, journal writing is a wonderful tool for accessing your inner wisdom. Several years ago I adopted the practice of journal writing first thing upon arising in the morning. In the quiet of the early morning hours as the sun is rising, I sit and write a couple of pages in longhand, allowing whatever thoughts are flowing through my mind to flow through my hand and onto the paper. During this time, I am somewhere between the dream state I have just left and the dawning of the new day. Journal writing has become a form of meditation and processing that has resulted in significant changes in my emotional, physical, and spiritual well-being. Studies have shown that people who engage in journal writing on a regular basis enhance the functioning of their immune systems and are less prone to illness. I think of this type of journal writing as a method of purification. It is a practice that I have woven into my daily life that enhances my sense of well-being and prevents the build-up of toxic emotions.

While you don't have to adhere to a schedule to benefit from journal writing, it does help to set aside a regular time. Some people enjoy writing in the early morning hours, while others like to journal just before sleeping in order to process the day's events. Don't worry about grammar or punctuation—you'll more readily access feelings if you bypass the intellect. Don't try to write anything of importance, but instead allow the free flow of any thoughts or images that appear in your mind to be transferred to paper by your hand. It may take a few writing sessions to completely relax, but you'll soon discover the joys of the unique insights into the inner workings of your mind that appear when you allow your thoughts to flow freely onto the paper. As you continue in your process of journal writing, you will strengthen your connection to your inner wisdom, which will help to guide you toward a healthy, fulfilling, and joyful life.

Relaxation Exercises

Relaxation is a skill that can be learned, just as stressful patterns of behavior are learned responses. By practicing the following simple exercises, you can teach your body to relax by letting go of muscle tension and chronic ways of being that create stress. You can also foster a state of peaceful mental relaxation that will allow your mind to be calm and centered. Try the following exercises, and choose your favorites. You might find it helpful to tape the exercises, or to have a friend read them to you so that you can fully appreciate the experience.

Gentle Progressive Relaxation

Lie down in a comfortable position and close your eyes. Take a deep, easy breath, expanding your abdomen as you inhale. Exhale completely, allowing your abdomen to fall. Take a couple of easy breaths in this way, focusing on the rhythm of your breath. Become aware of your thoughts, and take another deep, easy breath. As you exhale, imagine that you are releasing any worries with your exhalation. Let all of your concerns go as you take this time for deep, healing relaxation.

Bring your attention to your feet. Notice how your feet and toes feel. Be exquisitely aware of your feet, the feeling of the air around your feet, and the feeling of the surface that your feet are resting on. Gently breathe into your feet and toes, and with your next exhalation, release any tension that you may be holding in your feet. Take a moment to appreciate how good it feels to relax your feet.

Move your attention to your lower legs, becoming aware of any tension in your calves. Inhale, breathing into the tension, and as you exhale, imagine the tension flowing out of your lower legs. Bring your attention to your upper legs, noticing any tension that you are holding in your thighs. Breathe into the tension, and release it with your next exhalation. Take another deep, easy breath, and feel the tension flowing out of your thighs, down your calves, and out of your feet with your exhalation. Enjoy the deep feeling of relaxation that comes with the release of tension.

Feel your hips and buttocks resting against the surface that you are lying on. Take a deep, relaxing breath, and breathe into any tension there. As you exhale, let the tension flow out of your hips and buttocks. Move your attention to your lower back, and become aware of any tension that you are holding. Inhale deeply and easily into your lower back, and release any tightness with your exhalation. Take another deep breath, and let any remaining tension in your lower back, hips, buttocks, thighs, calves, and feet flow out of your body with your exhalation.

Move your attention to your shoulders, and become aware of any tension that you are holding in your shoulders. Breathe into the tension, and as you exhale, release the tension with your exhalation. Focus on your upper arms and any tension there. With your next exhalation, let go of tightness in your upper arms. Notice any tension in your lower arms and hands, and breathe out the tightness as you exhale. Gently expand your attention to include your shoulders, upper arms, lower arms, and hands, and become aware of any residual tension there. Inhale, and as you exhale, let go of any last bits of tension.

Bring your attention to your upper back, neck, and head. Feel the surface that your head and upper back are resting on. Become aware of any tension that you are holding in these areas, and breathe into the tightness. As you exhale, feel the tension flowing out of your scalp, your face, your neck, and your upper back. Take another deep, relaxing breath, and let go of any residual tension. Notice any tightness in your forehead and your eyes, and release the tension as you exhale. Let your attention move gently to your jaw and mouth, and inhale into the tension that you find there. Exhale, and relax your mouth and jaw completely. Take another deep inhalation, and release any remaining tension in your scalp, face, head, and neck.

Move your attention to your chest, and notice the gentle movement of your chest as you inhale. Exhale, and let any tension flow out of your chest. Let your attention move to your abdomen, and notice how your abdomen expands as you inhale. Exhale, and release any tightness in your abdominal area. Take another deep, relaxing breath, and let go of any last bits of tension in your chest and abdomen. Take a moment to gently scan your body, and if you find any pockets of residual tightness, breathe into that area, and let the tension go with your exhalation.

Continue breathing in a relaxed and easy manner for a few minutes, enjoying the deep sense of peace and relaxation that comes from letting go of tension. When you are ready, inhale deeply, stretch, and gently open your eyes as you return to a state of full alertness.

Palming

This simple exercise has profound relaxing and restorative effects on not only the eyes, but the entire body. Your eyes rarely have a chance to rest, except when you are sleeping. Palming refreshes your eyes and calms your mind, which helps to relax your entire body. Take a few moments throughout the day at various times to practice this exercise.

Sit comfortably, with your feet flat on the floor and your spine erect. If desired, rest your elbows on a table or desk, using a book or pillow to raise your elbows so that you can keep your spine erect and not lower your head. Rub your palms together briskly until they feel warm. Cup your palms so that your fingers do not touch your eyes, and place them at a slight angle over your eyes, crossing your fingers on the bridge of your nose and your forehead. Adjust your palms to create complete darkness. Close your eyes, and allow the velvety blackness to soothe your eyes.

Breathe deeply and rhythmically, imagining that your breath is circulating behind your eyes and carrying away tension. Relax your mind, and let any tension go with each exhalation. Keep your spine erect to allow the energy to flow freely throughout your head and neck. Continue breathing in a relaxed and easy manner for several minutes, or as long as you wish.

Relaxation with Music

Listening to music is a delightful method of relaxation therapy. Music can evoke deep feelings of calm, helping to ease tense muscles and soothe a tumultuous mind. Of course, it's important to choose the right music. Select pieces that you find especially soothing, and begin to create a collection specifically designed for healing relaxation. Try classical, instrumental, or chants—whatever evokes a sense of calm and well-being for you. Many selections in the New Age section of music and bookstores are especially created to calm the body and the mind.

Set aside 20 or 30 minutes for your music relaxation experience. Lie on the floor or sit in a comfortable chair and close your eyes. Breathe deeply and gently scan your body, exhaling and letting go of any tension that you find. Allow the music to flow around you and through you, filling you with peaceful harmonies. Focus your full attention on the music and release any thoughts that intrude by gently bringing your awareness back to the music. When the music ends, sit or lie quietly for a few moments and appreciate the deep feeling of relaxation that you have experienced.

Meditation

Meditation has been practiced for centuries in many spiritual traditions as a way of purifying the mind. Basically, meditation involves quieting the mind so that the mental chatter that fills your waking consciousness can be stilled, if even for a moment. Through quieting the mind, you cultivate a sense of calm, and come to know yourself in a deeper way. Meditation helps you to become aware of habitual patterns of thinking so that you can make better choices about how you are living. Meditation is an excellent way of relieving stress, because when the mind is calm, the body naturally follows. Many people experience feelings of deep peace and clarity through meditation. Experiment with the different meditation techniques that follow and find those which appeal to you.

For all forms of meditation, there are a few guidelines that will help to make your experience more fulfilling. Find a quiet place where you will not be disturbed. Wear loose, comfortable clothing, and sit on a pillow or in a comfortable chair that allows you to keep your spine upright. If you are sitting on the floor, cross your legs in a comfortable position. It helps to keep your spine erect if you sit on the edge of a firm cushion. If you are sitting in a chair, place your feet flat on the floor and sit upright, away from the back of the chair. You can place a firm pillow behind your lower back if necessary for support.

Practice meditation on an empty stomach, or at least 1 hour after a meal. Rest your hands comfortably on your thighs or in your lap. For most meditation practices, gently close your eyes to help to focus your attention inward. Begin each meditation with a couple of deep cleansing breaths to release any tension from your body. Plan to meditate for 20 to 30 minutes at a time, and establish a regular time and place for your meditation practice. You will enjoy the greatest benefits from meditation when you make it a regular part of your daily life.

Meditation on the Breath

Find a quiet place where you will not be disturbed, and sit in a comfortable position. Close your eyes, and begin by taking three deep, easy cleansing breaths to relax your body, exhaling slowly and completely through your slightly opened mouth. Relax into your normal breathing pattern, inhaling and exhaling through your nose. Focus your attention in a gentle way on your breathing. Just observe your breathing, without trying to change it in any way. When your attention wanders, gently bring it back to observing your breath. You will notice that your breathing will fall into an easy, natural rhythm. By focusing on your breath, you cleanse your mind of thoughts and allow your body to come into a deep state of healing quiet. Continue in this way for 20 minutes. When you are finished with your meditation, expand your attention to include your surroundings, and gently open your eyes.

Meditation on a Mantra

A mantra is simply a word or phrase that you repeat over and over to give your mind a peaceful focus. Choose a word or phrase that has meaning for you. It can be as simple as "peace" or "calm." Sit in a comfortable position, close your eyes, and take 3 slow, deep cleansing breaths, exhaling completely. Focus your attention on your mantra, and repeat the word over and over in your mind. Breathe normally, and synchronize your mantra with your breathing by repeating it on each exhalation. When your mind wanders, gently bring your attention back to your mantra. Continue your meditation for 20 minutes. Sit quietly for a few minutes at the end of your meditation, and then open your eyes.

Once you have chosen your mantra, stick with it. The word will become associated with the feelings you experience during meditation, and you will be able to elicit a deep sense of calm at any time by recalling your mantra.

Candle-Gazing Meditation

The simple act of gazing into a candle flame offers another meditation method for quieting the thoughts. Candle gazing provides a specific visual focus that helps to center the mind. Place a lighted candle 3 feet in front of you. Sit in a comfortable position with your spine erect and take 3 deep, slow cleansing breaths. Gently focus your attention on the candle. Center your attention on the flame, being aware of the color and shape of the flame, watching its every movement. After gazing at the candle for several minutes in this way, gently close your eyes. You will be able to see the image of the candle flame with your eyes shut. Continue to focus on the image, keeping your eyes gently closed. When the image fades into blackness, open your eyes and gaze at the candle again. Repeat the sequence 2 or 3 times, as desired.

Moving Meditation

Bringing your complete awareness to a task such as bathing, cooking, or washing the dishes allows you to bring the principles of meditation into your everyday life. Simply focus your attention completely on the task at hand. Slow your movements down to about half the speed at which you would normally move. Pay exquisite attention to your body, to each movement, to any feelings of tension or discomfort. Breathe into any tightness that you discover and consciously release the tension.

We often habitually perform the simplest tasks with much more effort than is called for. By paying close attention to your movements, you can learn to do whatever you need to do with the least expenditure of effort necessary. This will help your body to function optimally, and will leave you feeling relaxed and energized. Even a few minutes of moving meditation is refreshing for the body and mind, and provides a new perspective on the task at hand.

Healing Visualization

Visualization uses the power of your imagination to evoke changes in your mind or body. When you create a mental image of what you would like to manifest, your mind and body respond to the picture as though it were a real experience. Visualization can improve your health and can help you to replace negative habits with positive, life-affirming ones. Every action you take begins with a thought and an image in your mind. Relaxation and meditation help you to bring your thoughts and images into conscious awareness, and visualization ensures that you are creating the life that you truly desire! You may wish to have a friend read the following exercise to you, or you can record it onto a tape.

Lie in a comfortable position with your eyes closed. Take a deep, easy breath, and begin to relax your body and your mind. Focus your attention on your breath, noticing the rising and falling of your breath as it enters and leaves your body. Mentally direct your body to relax, from your toes to your scalp. Without effort, scan your body for tension. Breathe into any tightness that you find and release it with your exhalation.

Now imagine in your mind's eye a blank screen. Inhale, and visualize the number 5 on the screen. See the number 5 clearly in your mind. As you exhale, visualize the number 5 fading, and as you take a deep, relaxing inhalation, see the number 4 appear on the screen in your mind. Exhale, and allow the 4 to fade, and as you inhale again, see the number 3 appear on the screen. Notice how relaxed you are feeling, as you exhale and watch the number 3 fade. Inhale, and visualize the number 2 on the screen. Exhale, watching the number 2 fade, and allow yourself to become even more deeply relaxed. Inhale, and see the number 1 appear on the screen. Allow yourself to exhale completely, and watch the number 1 fade, leaving the screen blank.

Now watch the screen as an image begins to appear. See yourself on the screen, lying comfortably in a beautiful meadow. It's a warm, sunny day, and you are completely safe and protected. Feel the warmth of the sunlight on your body and the gentle breeze caressing your skin. See the rich green of the velvety grass, the deep azure blue of the sky, the white puffy clouds floating effortlessly above you. Smell the sweet freshness of the meadow grasses and flowers, and hear the pleasing sounds of the rustle of leaves in the breeze, the faint chirping of birds in the trees, and the melody of a gentle nearby stream. Allow yourself to sink even more deeply into this peaceful place, knowing that you are safe and protected. You are warm, comfortable, and completely safe.

Feel the warmth of the sun, and as you inhale, imagine that your body is filled with the golden healing light of the sun. Imagine every cell and organ of your body being bathed, purified, and healed by this warm, soothing light. Notice any place where the energy seems to get stuck, and breathe into it, using your breath and the purifying light to gently dissolve the blockage. Allow the healing energy of the golden light to flow freely throughout your body. Take a few minutes to scan your entire body, inhaling healing golden light and exhaling tension. Visualize your organs working in perfect harmony, and see yourself in vibrant health. Acknowledge the deep state of relaxation and well-being that you are experiencing, and know that you can access this state at any time. Relax in this place of well-being for a couple of minutes, enjoying the feeling of perfect health.

When you are ready, take a deep breath, and begin to slowly bring your attention back to the present moment. Become aware of your surroundings, stretch your arms and legs and gently open your eyes, while still maintaining a feeling of deep calmness and well-being.

A Compendium
of Purifying Herbs

The following herbs have been used for hundreds of years for cleansing and purification. As herbalism continues to enjoy a renaissance of interest, research studies are supporting the wisdom of the ancients who discovered the healing properties of these plants through many centuries of use and experimentation. Some of these herbs—garlic and ginger, for example—have been studied extensively, and science bears out their remarkable healing and detoxifying benefits. Not all these herbs have been proven by science to have the benefits ascribed to them—most have not even been studied in such a way. But centuries of use by wise people all over the world indicates that there is a good reason that they have enjoyed a place in the repertoire of herbal healers for all this time. Experiment with the herbs that appeal to you, and judge the benefits for yourself. Above all, listen to your intuition and strengthen your own inner healing wisdom.

Guidelines for Safety in Using Herbs

1. Use caution if you have a chronic disease. Cleansing herbs can often be helpful as part of a treatment program for chronic disease, but check with your health practitioner before beginning an herbal or any other type of cleansing program.

2. Women who are pregnant or nursing should not undergo a cleansing program. However, many herbs are safe to use during pregnancy and can ease uncomfortable symptoms such as nausea, constipation, and fatigue. Consult with your health care practitioner before using herbs in medicinal amounts, and avoid herbs which have uterine stimulating properties, such as goldenseal.

3. If you develop an unpleasant reaction to any herb you are taking, stop using the herb. Such reactions include nausea, diarrhea, or headache, and will generally occur within a couple of hours of taking the herb.

4. If you are over 65 or sensitive to foods or drugs, use lesser amounts of herbal preparations. Begin with half the recommended dosage and evaluate your response to the herb before increasing to the recommended amount.

5. Do not give medicinal amounts of herbs to children under the age of 2 without the supervision of your health care practitioner. Herbs can be wonderful for children, but infants should be given very small amounts and only with the okay from your health practitioner.

6. Everyone is different, but in general, use only the recommended amounts of herbs for the recommended length of time. More is not necessarily better. Some perfectly safe herbs can cause problems if taken in excess.

7. Develop your intuition when using herbs. After all, you know your body better than anyone else. The more attuned you are to the inner workings of your body, the healthier you will be. Understanding your body begins with paying attention. Listen, and your body will tell you what feels good, and what doesn't.

8. Always buy good quality herbs from a reputable source. Herbs, especially expensive ones like goldenseal, are sometimes adulterated with less costly and sometimes harmful herbs. This does not happen often, but to be safe, know your herb source.

9. Essential oils are highly concentrated and should never be used internally without the guidance of your health care practitioner.

Alfalfa (*Medicago sativa*)

Part used: *Leaves*

Alfalfa was used by the ancient Chinese to treat digestive problems and to stimulate the appetite. In ancient India, Ayurvedic physicians used alfalfa to treat fluid retention, arthritis, and ulcers. Alfalfa is rich in cleansing chlorophyll. Research has shown that it helps to lower blood cholesterol levels and even helps to cleanse cholesterol from the arteries. Alfalfa also helps the body to eliminate carcinogens by neutralizing and binding them in the intestine. Do not eat alfalfa seeds, or for that matter, alfalfa sprouts. The seeds contain a toxic amino acid called *canavanine*. Large amounts of canavanine may cause a blood-clotting disorder and interfere with the activity of white blood cells. Alfalfa leaves, however, are safe.

Make an infusion of alfalfa by steeping 1 to 2 teaspoons of the dried herb in 1 cup of boiling water for 10 to 15 minutes. Strain, and drink up to 3 cups a day. Alfalfa has a haylike, slightly bitter taste. Combine with peppermint to improve the flavor.

Aloe (*Aloe vera*)

Parts used: *The gel found in the leaves and the bitter juice (latex) extracted from the inner skin of the leaf*

The healing properties of aloe have been recognized since the time of the ancient Egyptians, who used it for treating infections and skin problems, and as a laxative. Traditional Chinese and Ayurvedic physicians prescribed aloe for intestinal worms, skin disorders, and menstrual problems, and the Greeks and Romans used aloe for burns, wounds, hemorrhoids, and ulcers.

Aloe vera gel applied externally is excellent for treating wounds, burns, and rashes, and is most effective when applied fresh from a sliced leaf. Aloe has been found to have antibacterial and antifungal activity against microorganisms such as *Candida albicans* and *E. coli*. In addition, aloe has anti-inflammatory properties which are useful both internally and externally, and it contains vitamin C, vitamin E, and zinc, all of which promote healing. Fresh aloe vera gel has been shown to stimulate the formation of connective tissue and the growth and repair of skin cells.

Internally, aloe vera gel or juice is helpful for constipation, peptic ulcers, and as a tonic to enhance immune functioning. Aloe improves the digestion of proteins and the assimilation of nutrients. The antibacterial properties of aloe also help to restore the intestinal tract to a healthy state by reducing the putrefaction of intestinal bacteria and limiting the growth of problem causing organisms such as *Candida albicans*.

The aloe latex, available as a powder or in tablet form, contains powerful laxative chemicals called *anthraquinones* that are strong purgatives. Aloe latex is the strongest of all the anthraquinone-containing herbs (others are *senna, buckthorn, cascara sagrada,* and *rhubarb*) and can cause severe intestinal cramping and diarrhea. For this reason, aloe latex is not recommended as a laxative, and other less drastically acting herbs such as cascara sagrada should be used instead. Aloe latex should definitely not be used by anyone with gastrointestinal problems such as irritable bowel syndrome, diverticulitis, or diverticulosis, and should not be used as a laxative by pregnant women because it may stimulate uterine contractions.

In Ayurvedic medicine, aloe vera gel is considered one of the primary rejuvenative tonics for the liver and spleen and for the female reproductive system. Aloe is rich in enzymes, and is used to stimulate digestive enzymes and to promote healthy digestion. As a tonic, take 2 teaspoons of aloe vera gel in water or juice or 1/4 cup of aloe vera juice with a pinch of turmeric or ginger once or twice daily.

Barberry (*Berberis vulgaris*)

Part used: Root bark

Barberry contains a powerful natural antibiotic called *berberine*, the same active ingredient that is found in goldenseal. The antibiotic properties were recognized long ago, as barberry root was used by the ancient Egyptians to prevent plagues, and by Ayurvedic physicians in India to treat dysentery. During the Middle Ages, barberry was used to treat liver and gallbladder diseases. Studies have proven the antibiotic properties of barberry. It has been shown to be effective against a wide range of microorganisms, including those that cause wound infections, diarrhea, urinary tract infections, and vaginal yeast infections. In addition to killing microorganisms, barberry also helps to stimulate the immune system by increasing the activity of *macrophages*, the white blood cells that consume harmful microorganisms and other cellular wastes.

Barberry has a bitter taste, which stimulates the flow of bile and helps to improve liver function. It is a mild and excellent liver tonic, and because of its blood-cleansing properties, is often prescribed as an herb for treating skin problems such as acne and boils. The bitter taste stimulates digestion and also has mild laxative action.

To make a decoction, simmer 1 teaspoon of barberry root in 1 cup of water for 20 minutes. Strain and drink up to 3 cups a day. Because berberine may stimulate the uterus, pregnant women should not take barberry.

Black Pepper (*Piper nigrum*)

Part used: *Fruit*

Black pepper is a good example of a healing herb that has found its way into the kitchen as a common culinary spice. In Ayurvedic medicine, black pepper is considered to be one of the most powerful digestive stimulants. It is prescribed to cleanse the gastrointestinal tract and to burn up *ama*, the toxins that accumulate in the digestive organs. Black pepper is recommended in Ayurvedic medicine as a digestive stimulant to improve weak digestion, which manifests in symptoms such as gas and abdominal bloating. It is also helpful as an expectorant for treating colds and upper respiratory infections, because it eliminates excessive mucus in the lungs and sinuses and stimulates circulation.

To enhance digestion, add freshly ground black pepper liberally to foods. A digestive tonic similar to one prescribed in Ayurvedic medicine combines equal parts of dried black peppercorns, dried ginger root, and fennel seeds. Grind the herbs together into a powder, and mix with enough honey to form a paste. Take 1/2 teaspoon with a small amount of hot water three times a day. Do not use large amounts of black pepper if you suffer from any inflammatory conditions of the digestive organs, such as ulcers.

Buckthorn (*Rhamnus cathartica*)

Part used: *Bark*

The Latin name of buckthorn says it all—*cathartica*. Buckthorn is a laxative that was used by European herbalists in the 13th century, who believed that purging the body was the key to healing most ills. Buckthorn contains anthraquinones, natural chemicals that stimulate contractions of the large intestine and have a strong laxative effect. Gentler anthraquinone laxatives include cascara sagrada.

Buckthorn is a good laxative in cases of stubborn constipation. Make an infusion of 1/2 teaspoon each of dried buckthorn bark and fennel seeds in 1 cup boiling water. Steep for 10 minutes, and drink before bed. It takes approximately 12 hours to take effect, so be patient and do not exceed the recommended dosage. Buckthorn can cause diarrhea and severe intestinal cramps if taken in excess. It should not be used by people with chronic gastrointestinal problems such as ulcers or colitis.

Burdock (*Articum lappa*)

Part used: *Root*

Burdock has a reputation as a gentle yet effective detoxifying herb. The rich concentration of minerals and other nutrients found in burdock root make it an excellent choice as part of a long-term cleansing program. Burdock's mild diuretic and laxative properties help rid body tissues of toxins, and at the same time, the nutritive components help to build healthy blood.

Burdock has been used for centuries in many healing traditions as a remedy for a variety of diseases. In Chinese and Ayurvedic medicine, burdock is prescribed to relieve colds and flus. In Western herbalism, burdock root is frequently recommended for treating skin problems such as acne, eczema, dandruff, and psoriasis. Natural antimicrobial constituents found in burdock root help to purify the blood, promoting the healing of skin problems such as boils and acne. The combined antimicrobial and diuretic properties of burdock are helpful for urinary tract infections.

The slightly bitter taste of burdock root stimulates the secretion of bile and promotes the flow of digestive juices, which improves the digestion and assimilation of nutrients. Because it improves digestive and eliminative functions and blood quality, burdock is often included as part of a comprehensive treatment program for degenerative diseases such as arthritis and cancer.

When brewed as a tea, burdock root has a slightly sweet, bitter, earthy taste. Burdock is also available fresh in many markets, and has a sweet, nutty flavor. To use the fresh root, scrub it well, slice into 1/4 to 1/2 inch rounds, and add to soups or stews. Simmer for approximately 30 minutes, or until tender. To use as a tea, prepare a decoction of the root by simmering 1 teaspoon of dried burdock root (or 2 teaspoons of fresh) in 1 cup of water for 20 minutes. Drink 3 to 4 cups throughout the day. Burdock combines well with other liver-cleansing herbs such as Oregon grape root, dandelion root, sarsaparilla, yellow dock, licorice root, and ginger root.

Cascara Sagrada (*Rhamnus purshiana*)

Part used: *Dried, aged bark*

Cascara sagrada was reverently known as the "sacred bark" to the Spanish explorers who came to Northern California. Like many travelers throughout the centuries, they suffered from a common problem—constipation. The native Indians introduced them to a tea made from the dried, aged bark of the cascara sagrada tree. Because of its effectiveness as a laxative, cascara sagrada has become one of the most popular herbal medicines in the world.

Cascara contains natural chemicals called anthraquinones that stimulate intestinal contractions. It has a milder action than other anthraquinone-containing laxatives such as aloe vera, buckthorn, senna, and rhubarb, and should be used first when an herbal laxative is needed. Cascara sagrada is helpful in cases of chronic constipation because it helps to restore intestinal tone. It encourages peristalsis and helps strengthen the muscles of the colon when they have become too relaxed. Cascara sagrada stimulates secretions throughout the entire digestive system, including the liver, gallbladder, pancreas, and stomach.

Infuse 1 to 2 teaspoons of dried bark in 1 cup of boiling water for 20 minutes. Adding 1/2 teaspoon of a carminative herb such as ginger or fennel will improve the taste and will help to prevent any possible cramping for those with especially sensitive digestive tracts. Drink 1 cup before bed, and another in the morning if needed. Or take 1/2 teaspoon of tincture in a small amount of hot water or ginger tea.

Cinnamon (*Cinnamomum zeylanicum*)

Part used: *Dried inner bark*

Cinnamon is one of the most popular spices in the kitchen, and because of its warming and stimulating properties, is a helpful digestive aid. Cinnamon was used by ancient Chinese and Ayurvedic herbalists as a treatment for diarrhea, indigestion, fever, and menstrual problems.

Cinnamon has potent antiseptic properties and has been found to kill microorganisms such as bacteria, fungi, and viruses, including *E. coli*, the cause of most urinary tract infections, and *Candida albicans*, the cause of vaginal yeast infections. Whole sticks of cinnamon bark are an excellent addition to a bitters digestive formula, or to a laxative or liver-cleansing formula. Cinnamon has *carminative* properties, which means that it helps to relieve gas and intestinal cramping. To make a sweet and spicy tea, add 1/2 teaspoon of powdered cinnamon to 1 cup of boiling water.

Cleavers (*Galium aparine*)

Parts used: *Aerial parts*

Cleavers is regarded as one of the best tonic herbs for the lymphatic system. It has *alterative*, or blood purifying, and diuretic properties. Cleavers is often prescribed for lymphatic swelling, including tonsillitis, and for skin problems such as psoriasis and eczema. It is also helpful for urinary tract infections, where it is combined with herbs that have demulcent, soothing properties such as marshmallow root and corn silk. Cleavers has a long history of use for the treatment of tumors, probably because it promotes lymphatic drainage and thus helps to cleanse the tissues.

Cleavers (also called *bedstraw*) is a common weed, and can be taken fresh from the yard and made into a tea. It has a pleasantly green, astringent taste. To make an infusion, steep 2 teaspoons of the dried herb or 2 tablespoons of chopped fresh plant in 1 cup of boiling water for 10 minutes. Drink 3 cups daily.

Clove (*Syzgium aromaticum*)

Parts used: *Dried flower buds*

Cloves are the buds of a tropical evergreen tree. They are used by traditional Chinese physicians to treat indigestion, diarrhea, and fungal infections, and by Ayurvedic physicians for respiratory and digestive problems. European herbalists use cloves for treating indigestion, nausea, diarrhea, intestinal worms, and coughs. The aromatic essential oils in cloves help to relax the digestive tract and relieve intestinal gas. Cloves also have antimicrobial properties, and are effective against fungi and bacteria as well as intestinal parasites.

To make an infusion, steep 1 teaspoon of dried cloves in 1 cup of boiling water for 15 minutes. Strain, and drink up to 3 cups a day.

Corn Silk (*Zea mays*)

Parts used: *Stigmas from female flowers*

Corn silk has soothing, gentle diuretic properties that make it effective for cleansing the urinary tract. Corn silk helps to buffer the effects of stronger, potentially irritating diuretic herbs such as juniper berries.

Save the corn silk from fresh organic corn and use it fresh for tea, or dry it for later use. To make a tea from corn silk, pour 1 cup of boiling water over 2 teaspoons of dried corn silk or 1 to 2 tablespoons of fresh corn silk and steep for 10 to 15 minutes. Strain, and drink up to 3 cups a day.

Dandelion (*Taraxacum officinale*)

Parts used: *Root and leaf*

When you think of dandelion, your first thought might be of the tenacious weed that crops up in your lawn despite your best efforts to eradicate it. But when you discover the healing benefits of this humble little plant, you might turn your efforts to cultivating dandelions instead.

Dandelion has a long history of use in folk medicine throughout the world. In Europe, dandelion has been used for treating skin problems, liver sluggishness, digestive disturbances, and fluid retention. The Chinese have used dandelion for treating colds, skin diseases, obesity, liver disease, and digestive ailments. In most other parts of the world, the use of dandelion has focused primarily on the liver.

Dandelion root is one of the best herbs for cleansing the liver. The moderately bitter-tasting root stimulates digestive secretions and promotes healthy digestion. Not only does dandelion promote the flow of salivary and gastric juices, but it also stimulates the release of bile by the liver and gallbladder. Studies have shown that dandelion is helpful for treating problems such as liver congestion, hepatitis, gallstones, jaundice, and bile duct inflammation. Because of its actions on the liver, dandelion has gentle laxative effects.

Dandelion leaf is a highly effective and safe diuretic herb. It is especially useful in cases of water retention, as for example, the bloating associated with PMS. Dandelion leaf is comparable in effectiveness to pharmaceutical diuretics, but without the harmful side effects. Synthetic diuretics cause the body to eliminate potassium and can cause dangerous problems such as heart rhythm disturbances. Dandelion leaf is rich in potassium, which helps to replace the potassium that is lost through increased urination.

Dandelion is a nutritive herb as well as a cleansing herb. It is high in beta carotene and vitamin C, iron, calcium, magnesium, potassium, and other trace minerals. Dandelion greens are the richest source of beta carotene of all greens. Just one cup of fresh dandelion greens contains between 7,000 and 13,000 I.U. of beta carotene. If you have a chemical-free lawn, let the dandelions grow and pick the young greens early in the spring. Avoid using the mature leaves, which become unpleasantly bitter. When young and tender, dandelion leaves are delicious included in salads, soups, and sautés. You can also plant dandelion greens in your garden to include in your meals year-round.

Dandelion is extremely safe and is considered nontoxic, even in large amounts. Dandelion root tea has an earthy, sweet, and slightly bitter flavor and is appropriate to use as a general herbal tonic and to improve liver function. To make a decoction, simmer 2 teaspoons of dried chopped root in 1 cup of water for 15 minutes. Strain, and drink 3 cups daily. For a leaf infusion to relieve water retention, add

2 teaspoons of dried leaves to 1 cup of boiling water and steep for 10 minutes. Strain, and drink 3 cups daily.

Echinacea (*Echinacea angustifolia, Echinacea purpurea*)

Parts used: *Root, flowers, stems and leaves*

Echinacea is native to the plains of North America and was the primary medicine used by the Plains Indians. They used echinacea root to treat wounds, including snakebites, and drank echinacea tea as a remedy for colds, infectious diseases such as smallpox, and arthritis. Echinacea was adopted by the settlers and was widely used during epidemics. It became a popular blood-purifying remedy, and was used to treat all kinds of illnesses, including wounds and blood poisoning, and infectious diseases such as influenza, chicken pox, meningitis, and malaria.

Echinacea is an excellent herbal antibiotic and has immune-stimulating properties. It contains a natural antibiotic called *echinacoside* which kills a wide range of microorganisms, including viruses, bacteria, fungi, and protozoa. Echinacea increases the production of T-lymphocytes, infection-fighting white blood cells, and also enhances the activity of macrophages, white blood cells that engulf and destroy trouble-causing microorganisms, tumor cells, and cellular debris. Echinacea also strengthens cells against invading microorganisms, and increases the activity of natural killer cells, another type of white blood cell that destroys cells that have become cancerous or infected with viruses. Herbalists and health practitioners prescribe echinacea as a treatment for colds and flus and other upper respiratory infections, urinary tract infections, and boils and other indications of impure blood. Echinacea has been shown to have anti-inflammatory properties and to stimulate tissue regeneration, which supports its use as a wound healer. Because of its ability to cleanse harmful microorganisms from the body, echinacea is a valuable addition to a cleansing program.

Echinacea has a bitter, slightly sweet flavor. To make a decoction, simmer 2 teaspoons of echinacea root in 1 cup of water for 15 minutes. Strain, and drink up to 3 cups a day. In tincture form, take up to 1 teaspoon 3 times daily.

Elder (*Sambucus nigra*)

Part used: *Flowers*

Elder is an excellent diaphoretic herb, and assists the body in eliminating toxins through the skin by promoting perspiration. The flowers help to reduce mucus congestion in the respiratory tract. They also have gentle diuretic properties, and help to eliminate toxins via the kidneys.

Elder flowers have a slightly bitter, sweet flavor. Combine with peppermint and yarrow for an effective cleansing tea that is especially useful for relieving cold and flu symptoms and will help to naturally bring down a fever by inducing sweating. To prepare as a tea, pour 1 cup of boiling water over 2 teaspoons of elder flowers and steep for 10 minutes. Strain, and drink up to 3 cups a day. When treating a cold or flu, elder tea is most effective when it is taken hot.

Eucalyptus (*Eucalyptus globulus*)

Part used: *Leaves*

The essential oil distilled from eucalyptus has been used since the 19th century as an antiseptic for wounds, and also as an inhalation for treating bronchial infections. Eucalptus oil gives mentholated chest rubs and cough drops their characteristic refreshing scent. Studies show that *eucalyptol*, the natural chemical in eucalyptus, effectively kills a variety of bacteria and viruses, and the potent essential oil found in eucalyptus helps to loosen mucus congestion.

Eucalyptus has a spicy, cool taste. To make a tea, steep 1 to 2 teaspoons of dried leaves in 1 cup of boiling water for 10 minutes. Strain, and drink up to 3 cups a day. To make an herbal steam inhalant to cleanse the lungs and sinuses and relieve respiratory infections, pour 1 1/2 quarts of boiling water over a large handful of eucalyptus leaves, cover, and steep for 10 minutes. Remove the lid, make a towel tent over your head and the pot of steaming water, and breathe in the steam for 10 minutes. Or simply add 2 drops of eucalyptus essential oil to a pot of hot water and inhale the fragrant steam. Eucalyptus essential oil can also be added to a massage oil blend or to a bath to stimulate circulation and to relieve sore muscles and joints. Use 10 drops per ounce of almond oil for a massage, or 7 drops in a tub of warm water for a bath.

Fennel (*Foeniculum vulgare*)

Part used: *Seeds*

Fennel has traditionally been used for centuries as a digestive aid in China, India, and Europe. The aromatic essential oils in fennel have antispasmodic properties and help to relax the digestive tract. Fennel also helps to relieve intestinal gas. In Europe, fennel is used as a treatment for indigestion and colic. Ayurvedic practitioners regard fennel seeds as one of the best herbs for digestion. They prescribe fennel to strengthen *agni*, the digestive fire, and to alleviate gastrointestinal discomfort. In addition, fennel seeds are believed to calm the nerves and to promote mental clarity.

Ayurvedic practitioners recommend lightly roasting fennel seeds in a dry skillet to release the essential oils. Take 1 teaspoon after meals, chewed well, to relieve indigestion. To make a pleasant, licorice flavored infusion, steep 1 to 2 teaspoons of lightly crushed seeds in 1 cup of boiling water for 10 minutes. Strain, and drink up to 3 cups a day. To promote healthy digestion, drink 1/2 cup of warm fennel tea 1/2 hour before meals, and 1/2 cup after. Fennel is an excellent addition to a digestive bitters formula or to a laxative formula. The aromatic seeds help to soften the taste of some of the more bitter herbs while adding beneficial digestion-enhancing properties.

Fenugreek (*Trigonella foenum-graecum*)

Part used: *Seeds*

Fenugreek has been used since Egyptian times to treat respiratory and gastrointestinal problems. In Ayurvedic medicine, the seeds are used in cooking to enhance digestion. Fenugreek contains significant amounts of mucilage, which helps to soothe inflamed or irritated membranes throughout the body. It also has expectorant properties, and helps to loosen and eliminate excess mucus from the respiratory tract. As a warm tea, it soothes coughs and bronchitis. The bitter flavor of fenugreek promotes healthy digestion by stimulating the flow of bile. Studies have shown that fenugreek helps to lower levels of harmful LDL cholesterol.

To prepare a tea from fenugreek, simmer 1 to 2 teaspoons of the seeds in 1 cup of water for 10 minutes. Strain and drink up to 3 cups a day. Fenugreek has a bitter and sweet taste, and can be combined with fennel or anise to improve the flavor.

Garlic (*Allium sativum*)

Part used: *Bulb*

Garlic is perhaps the most beloved culinary herb, and is certainly one of the most versatile of the healing herbs. The pungent volatile sulphur compounds found in garlic contain a variety of healing properties. From early Egyptian times, garlic was valued for preventing illness and enhancing health. It was prescribed for a variety of illnesses, including menstrual problems, tumors, heart disease, and tapeworms. The great Greek physician Hippocrates recommended garlic for infections, cancer, and digestive problems, and Ayurvedic physicians used garlic to treat cancer and leprosy. During World War I, garlic was used by the British, French, and Russians to treat infections, and garlic was also used extensively by the Russians in World War II in lieu of penicillin. Numerous research studies have upheld the traditional use of garlic as an herbal antibiotic. Raw garlic contains a natural substance called *alliin* which is transformed into the potent natural antibiotic *allicin* when it is chewed or chopped.

Garlic also has powerful healing effects on the cardiovascular system. It helps to reduce blood pressure, decrease cholesterol levels, and prevents the dangerous blood clots that can trigger heart attacks and strokes. Other research indicates that garlic provides potent protection against cancer. European researchers have shown that garlic helps to eliminate lead and other toxic heavy metals from the body.

The best way to take advantage of garlic's healing and cleansing properties is to use it liberally in cooking. Most of the healing benefits of garlic are unaffected by heat, but to access garlic's antibiotic properties, it must be eaten raw and either chopped or chewed. Try adding raw minced garlic to soups or pasta dishes just before serving. If garlic breath offends you (or someone you're close to) try chewing a breath-freshening herb such as parsley or fennel.

Gentian (*Gentiana lutea*)

Part used: *Root*

Gentian root has been valued for more than 3000 years as a digestive bitter, and is one of the strongest bitter herbs known. It was used by the ancient Egyptians, Greeks, and Romans to stimulate sluggish appetites, and to treat a variety of digestive disorders including intestinal worms and liver problems. In China, gentian is prescribed to treat digestive complaints, headaches, sore throats, and arthritis. Ayurvedic medicine also recommends gentian for liver and digestive disorders.

Gentian is excellent for treating general sluggishness of the digestive system. The root contains a substance called *gentianine* that stimulates the production of saliva, gastric and pancreatic digestive fluids, and bile. By improving digestion, gentian acts as a whole body strengthener. To take advantage of gentian's digestion-enhancing properties, the bitter taste must come into contact with the taste buds. The bitter flavor elicits a reflex action in the digestive tract that starts the flow of digestive enzymes and fluids.

To make a decoction, simmer 1 teaspoon of dried shredded root in 2 cups of water for 20 minutes. Allow to cool to room temperature and strain. To enhance digestion, take 1 tablespoon to 1/4 cup of tea 15 to 30 minutes before meals. Gentian is extremely bitter and may best be tolerated in tincture form. Take 1/2 teaspoon of tincture in a small amount of warm water or ginger tea 15 to 30 minutes before meals. Do not exceed the recommended dosage. Too much can irritate the stomach and cause nausea.

Ginger (*Zingiber officinale*)

Part used: *Root*

Ginger is a powerful tonic herb that offers healing benefits for almost every organ system of the body. The pungent essential oils found in ginger root are the source of ginger's healing properties. Ginger has a particular affinity for the digestive tract and has been used for centuries as a digestive aid in the Chinese, Ayurvedic, and European herbal traditions. It effectively relieves a wide variety of digestive ailments, including nausea, heartburn, flatulence, and diarrhea. Ginger has been found to alleviate the nausea of motion sickness better than Dramamine, the drug usually prescribed for the malady.

The antispasmodic and antiinflammatory properties of ginger not only soothe digestive upsets but also help to relieve menstrual cramps, migraine headaches, and arthritis. Ginger keeps the cardiovascular system healthy by reducing cholesterol levels, lowering blood pressure, and preventing the blood clots that lead to heart attacks and strokes. And studies have shown that ginger stimulates immune activity and helps to kill the influenza virus, making it especially helpful for treating colds and flus.

Ginger has been traditionally valued for its diaphoretic properties which makes it excellent for promoting the elimination of toxins through the skin. A cup of hot ginger tea is a delicious way to fight off colds and flus. Include ginger frequently in your meals to take advantage of its health benefits and delicious spicy taste. Scrub the root, but do not peel it, because many of the active properties are contained in the skin. Add thinly sliced ginger root to soups, pasta and rice dishes, salad dressings, and sautés.

To make ginger tea, simmer 2 teaspoons of fresh chopped ginger root in 1 cup of water in a covered pot for 5 minutes. Turn off the heat and allow to steep for an additional 5 minutes. Strain, and add honey if desired. Drink 3 to 4 cups daily. Ginger is often effective for relieving morning sickness during pregnancy. However, because it is also traditionally regarded as a menstruation promoter, pregnant women should consult their health care practitioners before using ginger.

Goldenseal (*Hydrastis canadensis*)

Parts used: *Rhizome and roots*

Goldenseal is a North American herb that was used by Native Americans for treating a variety of ailments, including respiratory, digestive, and genito-urinary tract infections as well as for eye and skin ailments. Goldenseal contains 2 powerful natural chemicals, *berberine* and *hydrastine*. Berberine is also found in barberry root and Oregon grape root. Berberine has direct antimicrobial action and kills harmful bacteria and yeast in the gastrointestinal tract. It is effective against a wide range of problem-causing microorganisms, including *staphylococcus, chlamydia, E. coli, salmonella, trichomonas, giardia,* and *Candida albicans*. In addition, berberine stimulates the immune system by increasing macrophage activity, the white blood cells that consume bacteria, viruses, and cancer cells. A strong tea can be used externally as an antiseptic for wounds and also as a topical treatment for eczema and fungal skin problems such as ringworm and athlete's foot.

Goldenseal helps to cleanse the blood and lymph by improving blood flow to the spleen and through stimulating macrophage activity. The bitter taste promotes the secretion of bile, thus improving liver function. These actions support the traditional use of goldenseal as a blood cleanser. Goldenseal also has anti-inflammatory and astringent properties, and helps to cleanse mucous membranes and lymph glands throughout the body.

To make an infusion, add 1/2 to 1 teaspoon of powdered root to 1 cup of boiling water. Steep 10 minutes and drink up to 2 cups a day. Goldenseal has a very bitter taste. In tincture form, take 1/2 to 1 teaspoon 3 times a day in a small amount of warm water. Pregnant women should not use goldenseal because it may cause uterine contractions. Hydrastine, a constituent of goldenseal, may raise blood pressure. Consult your health practitioner before using goldenseal if you have heart disease, high blood pressure, glaucoma, or diabetes.

Juniper Berries (*Juniperus communis*)

Part used: *Dried fruits*

The use of juniper dates back to the Egyptians, where it was used as a ceremonial cleansing herb and burned in temples for purification cermonies. When taken internally, juniper helps to cleanse the urinary tract by stimulating the flow of urine. Juniper berries contain an aromatic essential oil that is a natural diuretic chemical. The potent essential oils also have antimicrobial properties and are helpful for relieving urinary tract infections. Because of its diuretic properties, juniper can help to alleviate premenstrual water retention. Juniper also has anti-inflammatory properties and helps to cleanse acidic wastes from the bloodstream. In Europe, preparations of juniper are prescribed for treating arthritis and gout.

If used in excessive amounts or taken for a prolonged period of time, juniper can cause kidney irritation. Juniper should not be used by anyone with any type of kidney disease, including kidney infections, and should not be used during pregnancy. Avoid taking juniper for more than a couple of weeks at a time. Juniper berry tea has a pleasantly pungent, slightly sweet and bitter flavor. Make an infusion by steeping 1 teaspoon of the crushed dried berries in 1 cup of boiling water for 10 to 15 minutes. Drink up to 2 cups daily. Juniper combines well with other diuretic herbs such as cornsilk and marsh-mallow, which have soothing demulcent properties that help to buffer the strong action of juniper.

Juniper essential oil has stimulating properties and is considered one of the best remedies for cellulite. It is also helpful for muscle pains and arthritis. Never use juniper essential oil internally. For a bath, add 5 drops of juniper essential oil to 1 teaspoon of witch hazel and add to a tubful of hot water. For a massage oil, add 10 drops of juniper oil to 1 ounce of almond oil. Do not apply undiluted juniper essential oil directly to the skin, and do not use juniper oil during pregnancy or if you have kidney disease.

Licorice (*Glycyrrhiza glabra*)

Part used: Root

Licorice is one the primary healing herbs used in Chinese medicine, and is included in almost all Chinese herbal formulas to harmonize the action of other herbs. The demulcent, soothing properties of licorice are prescribed for alleviating respiratory, digestive, and urinary tract complaints. Licorice also has antimicrobial properties and enhances immune function, which makes it helpful for treating colds and flus. Licorice is beneficial when included in liver-cleansing formulas because it improves liver function by preventing free radical damage. In addition, licorice has anti-inflammatory properties, and appears to be beneficial for relieving arthritis symptoms.

In large doses, licorice may cause water retention. People with high blood pressure, cardiovascular or kidney disease should not use licorice without the supervision of a health practitioner.

Licorice has an extremely sweet taste, which makes it a welcome addition to herbs that have a less than pleasant flavor. It also makes a tasty tea on its own. To prepare licorice tea, simmer 1/2 to 1 teaspoon of licorice root in 1 cup of water for 10 minutes. Strain, and drink up to 3 cups a day.

Marshmallow (*Althaea officinalis*)

Part used: Root

Marshmallow has long been valued in European and Eastern herbal traditions for its soothing properties. It contains a large amount of mucilage, which is easily extracted in water and creates a slightly thick consistency when made into a tea. This soothing, slippery quality makes marshmallow excellent for treating any inflammatory condition, including gastrointestinal disorders such as ulcers, colitis, or acid stomach and respiratory problems such as bronchitis, sore throats, and coughs. Marshmallow also has gentle diuretic properties which make it helpful for relieving urinary tract infections. Marshmallow has also been shown in studies to have immune-enhancing properties, as well as mild laxative and expectorant action.

In Ayurvedic medicine, marshmallow is considered an excellent rejuvenative tonic because it moistens the tissues of the body. Marshmallow is a good addition to an herbal formula because it buffers the effects of stronger acting herbs, which reduces the possibility of irritation. Marshmallow has a pleasant, sweet flavor and can be added to any cleansing formula or made into a simple tea. To prepare marshmallow tea, simmer 1 teaspoon of chopped dried root in 1 cup of boiling water for 10 minutes. Let steep an additional 10 minutes, strain, and drink up to 3 cups a day.

Milk Thistle (*Silybum marianum*)

Part used: Seeds

Milk thistle contains natural compounds that are powerful antioxidants and provide potent protection for the liver. Researchers in Germany have found that milk thistle protects the liver from drug and heavy metal poisoning. It is even effective against the deadly Amanita mushroom, one of the most toxic liver substances known. Studies show that milk thistle not only protects the liver from damage by toxins, but also stimulates liver regeneration. In Europe, milk thistle is used as a liver tonic and is prescribed for treating serious liver diseases such as hepatitis and cirrhosis. Because it improves the ability of the liver to purify the blood, milk thistle has been found to be effective in treating skin diseases such as psoriasis. Milk thistle has also shown to be helpful in preventing or treating gallstones.

The active ingredient in milk thistle is *silymarin*, a potent antioxidant that prevents free radical damage and stimulates the growth of healthy new liver cells. Silymarin enhances the detoxification of harmful chemicals by increasing the glutathione content of the liver. *Glutathione* is an antioxidant produced by the body which is responsible for detoxifying hormones, drugs, and other chemicals.

Milk thistle is an excellent herb to include in any herbal cleansing program. Because the liver filters the blood, improving liver function is essential for detoxification. For treating chronic diseases such as hepatitis or cirrhosis, standardized extracts of milk thistle are usually recommended. The standard dosage is 140 milligrams of silymarin 3 times daily. For general cleansing and liver support, add milk thistle seeds to a liver-cleansing tea or tincture. The seeds have a hard coating and should be ground in a coffee grinder before using. To make an infusion from milk thistle, steep 1 teaspoonful of the ground seeds in 1 cup of boiling water for 15 minutes. Strain, and drink 3 cups a day. Milk thistle seeds can also be ground and added to cereals or sprinkled on salads.

Mullein (*Verbascum thapsus*)

Part used: *Leaves*

Mullein has been valued in a variety of herbal traditions for relieving respiratory complaints. Ayurvedic physicians in ancient India used mullein for the treatment of coughs, as did Native Americans. Mullein is rich in mucilage, which gives it soothing properties. It has expectorant action and helps to eliminate excess mucus from the respiratory tract. Mullein is excellent made into a tea for relieving coughs, bronchitis, and respiratory allergies. And mullein is also often recommended by herbalists as a lymphatic cleanser.

Mullein has a bitter flavor. To make a tea, pour 1 cup of boiling water over 1 to 2 teaspoons of dried mullein leaves and steep for 10 minutes. Strain, and drink up to 3 cups a day.

Nettle (*Urtica dioica*)

Part used: *Leaves*

In Europe, nettle leaves are commonly eaten in the early spring to cleanse and strengthen the blood. Nettle is rich in vitamins and minerals, including iron, calcium, magnesium, potassium, beta-carotene, and vitamin C. It also contains easily absorbable amino acids. The wealth of nutrients in nettle makes it an excellent energy-building tonic herb. In addition, nettle has diuretic and astringent properties and helps to eliminate excess fluids from body tissues. A warm infusion of nettle helps to relieve mucus congestion in the respiratory tract, while a cool infusion acts as a diuretic and soothing tea for the kidneys and bladder and is helpful for bladder infections. The diuretic properties of nettle also make it useful for relieving premenstrual water retention.

The common name for nettle is *stinging nettle*. If you can find fresh nettles, they make a delicious potherb. Nettle grows in rich soil in moist woodlands and near rivers and streams. Use a good plant identification book to help you identify nettle, and collect the fresh plant in the early spring, before it flowers. It may be irritating to the kidneys after flowering. The tiny hairs on the underside of the leaves and stem contain an irritant that causes intense stinging pain when touched. However, when nettles are cooked, the stinging juice is neutralized. Cook fresh nettles in a minimum of water by washing the leaves and placing the wet leaves in a heavy covered pot to steam for 5 minutes, or until the leaves are wilted. Season with lemon and olive oil.

Nettle tea can be enjoyed as a daily health tonic. To make an infusion, pour 1 cup of boiling water over 1 to 2 teaspoons of dried nettle, and steep for 10 minutes. Strain and drink up to 3 cups a day. Capsules of freeze-dried nettle have been found to be helpful for the symptomatic relief of hay fever. Take 2 capsules as needed to relieve symptoms.

Oregon Grape (*Mahonia aquifolium*)

Part used: *Root*

Oregon grape contains *berberine*, a powerful natural antibiotic that is also found in barberry and goldenseal. Oregon grape is traditionally used as a blood cleanser because of its action on the liver. It has bitter principles that stimulate the flow of bile, which cleanses the liver and acts as a mild natural laxative. Berberine also improves blood quality by increasing the flow of blood to the spleen, which filters the blood, and by stimulating the activity of white blood cells which consume and destroy bacteria, viruses, cancer cells, and other cellular wastes.

Because of its blood and liver cleansing actions, Oregon grape is often recommended for treating chronic skin conditions such as acne, psoriasis, and eczema. Oregon grape is excellent when included as part of a liver-cleansing formula during a detoxification program. It combines well with burdock root, yellow dock, sarsaparilla, ginger root, and licorice root. To make a tea from Oregon grape, simmer 1 to 2 teaspoons of dried root in 1 cup of water for 15 minutes. Strain, and drink up to 3 cups a day.

Parsley (*Petroselinum crispum*)

Part used: Leaves

Parsley was prescribed by ancient Roman physicians and European herbalists as a diuretic and was also eaten to freshen the breath. The essential oils found in parsley have mild laxative and diuretic properties. Because of its diuretic action, parsley is used in Europe to treat high blood pressure. Parsley tea can also help to relieve the uncomfortable bloating many women experience premenstrually. In addition, parsley acts as a gentle digestive aid and helps to relieve intestinal gas.

The dark green leaves of parsley are high in beta carotene and vitamin C and are one of the richest sources of chlorophyll, a natural breath freshener and blood purifier. Use parsley liberally during a cleansing program by adding the finely chopped leaves to soups and salads, and by juicing a handful of fresh parsley sprigs with carrots or beets for a cleansing juice cocktail. For a quick breath freshener, chew a sprig of parsley after a meal. Pregnant women should not use parsley medicinally because it can stimulate uterine contractions, but using moderate amounts of parsley in cooking is fine.

Parsley makes a fresh tasting, mildly spicy tea. Steep 1 tablespoon of chopped fresh parsley in 1 cup of boiling water for 10 minutes. Drink up to 3 cups daily.

Peppermint (*Mentha piperita*)

Parts used: Aerial parts

The ancient Egyptians used mint to soothe stomach upsets, and Chinese and Ayurvedic physicians have prescribed mint for centuries as a digestive aid and to relieve colds and fevers. Peppermint contains *menthol*, a potent essential oil that has antispasmodic, decongestant, and antimicrobial properties. The essential oils in peppermint help to relax the digestive tract, relieve indigestion and intestinal gas, and stimulate the flow of bile and digestive secretions. The antispasmodic properties also help to ease menstrual cramps and headaches.

Peppermint has diaphoretic properties which stimulate the release of toxins through perspiration and help to naturally lower fevers. As a hot tea or an herbal steam inhalation, peppermint relieves congestion by promoting the expulsion of mucus from the respiratory tract.

Peppermint has a cool, refreshing flavor. To make a tea, pour 1 cup of boiling water over 1 teaspoon of dried peppermint leaves and steep for 10 minutes. Strain, and drink up to 3 cups a day. To relieve cold and flu symptoms, combine peppermint with elder flower and yarrow and drink hot. For a steam inhalation to relieve respiratory congestion, pour 1 1/2 quarts of boiling water over 1 to 2 tablespoons of dried peppermint leaves. Let steep for 10 minutes in a covered pot. Uncover the pot, make a towel tent over your head and the steaming pot, and inhale the steam for 10 to 15 minutes.

Prickly Ash (*Zanthoxylum americanum*)

Part used: *Bark*

Prickly ash has circulation-stimulating properties and is traditionally used to improve blood and lymphatic flow. It also has diaphoretic action, which promotes cleansing by enhancing the elimination of toxins through the skin. Prickly ash is often recommended for chronic problems related to toxicity such as arthritis, rheumatism, and skin disorders and also for problems related to stagnant circulation such as varicose veins.

To make a tea from prickly ash, pour 1 cup of boiling water over 1 to 2 teaspoons of the bark and let steep for 15 minutes. Strain, and drink up to 3 cups a day.

Psyllium (*Plantago psyllium*)

Parts used: *Seeds, seed husks*

Psyllium is one of the safest and gentlest laxatives available and has been used by traditional Chinese and Ayurvedic physicians to treat constipation and diarrhea. Today, psyllium seeds are the primary ingredient in over-the-counter bulk-forming laxatives such as Metamucil. When added to water, psyllium seeds expand to more than 10 times their original size. This creates larger stools, which naturally stimulates peristalsis, the intestinal contractions that move wastes through the large intestine. By creating softer, bulkier stools, psyllium can help to relieve chronic gastrointestinal problems such as hemorrhoids and constipation. Psyllium is a rich source of soluble fiber, which absorbs toxins and excess cholesterol in the intestinal tract and helps to safely eliminate them from the body.

It is essential when taking psyllium to drink plenty of fluids— at least 1 full glass of water for each teaspoon of psyllium. Not drinking enough fluids with psyllium can create constipation instead of alleviating it. For treating constipation, take 1 teaspoon of psyllium seed husks in 1 glass of water 1 to 3 times daily. If you have a sensitive digestive tract, begin with 1/2 teaspoon and work your way up to the recommended dosage. Psyllium begins to thicken immediately when added to water, and if you wait more than a few seconds to drink it, it will become an undrinkable gel. Taking psyllium 15 to 30 minutes before meals acts as a natural appetite suppressant. In Ayurvedic medicine, psyllium seeds are believed to reduce *agni*, the digestive fire. To counteract this effect, take psyllium with a stimulating and warming digestive herbal tea made from ginger or fennel seeds.

Red Clover (*Trifolium pratense*)

Parts used: *Flower tops*

Red clover has long been used as an ingredient in cleansing and detoxification formulas, including formulas for herbal cancer treatments in many different cultures around the world. Researchers at the National Cancer Institute have found that red clover does contain anticancer compounds, including *genistein*, which has been found to repress the growth of all types of cancers. Red clover is also rich in antioxidants, which help to prevent the cellular damage that leads to cancer. It is considered a gentle but effective blood purifier, cleansing not only the blood but also the lymphatic system.

Red clover grows abundantly in open fields and lawns. If you choose to harvest your own, the blossoms should be picked when the flower heads are fully in bloom, in the late spring or early summer. Red clover makes a pleasantly sweet tea. Steep 1 to 2 teaspoons of dried flower tops in 1 cup of boiling water for 10 to 15 minutes. Strain, and drink up to 3 cups a day. Red clover is often combined with other blood-cleansing herbs such as burdock, yellow dock, and dandelion root.

Sarsaparilla (*Smilax officinalis*)

Parts used: *Root and rhizome*

Sarsaparilla has a long history of use as a blood purifier and is one of the classic liver tonic herbs. It was originally prescribed for the treatment of impure blood conditions by cultures as diverse as the Chinese and Europeans. Today, sarsaparilla is used for problems related to blood toxicity such as psoriasis and arthritis. In research studies, sarsaparilla has been shown to bind bacterial toxins in the gastrointestinal tract. If these toxins are absorbed into the bloodstream through the permeable intestinal wall, they can cause the inflammation and cell damage characteristic of many diseases such as arthritis and psoriasis. Sarsaparilla also has diuretic and diaphoretic properties, which promote the elimination of toxins through the urinary tract and the skin.

Make a decoction of sarsaparilla by simmering 1 to 2 teaspoons of dried root in 1 cup of boiling water for 15 minutes. Strain, and drink up to 3 cups a day. Sarsaparilla has a sweet, somewhat odd flavor. It combines well with other liver- and blood-cleansing herbs such as burdock, yellow dock, and dandelion root. Add good tasting herbs such as ginger and fennel to improve the taste.

Senna (*Cassia senna*)

Part used: *Dried fruit pods*

Senna has been used for centuries as a laxative, and is included in a number of over-the-counter laxative preparations. It contains the same natural chemicals found in cascara sagrada, aloe vera, and buckthorn that stimulate peristalsis, the wavelike contractions that move wastes through the intestinal tract. Senna has a stronger action than cascara sagrada, and can cause intestinal cramps, diarrhea, and nausea. It should only be used as a last resort for treating constipation. Bulk laxatives, such as psyllium, should be used first, as well as more gentle laxative herbs such as yellow dock and cascara sagrada.

Because of senna's powerful cathartic properties, it should not be used by pregnant women or nursing mothers or people who have irritable bowel syndrome or hemorrhoids. Senna has an unpleasant taste, and is best tolerated in tincture form. Take 1/2 to 1 teaspoon of tincture in a small amount of warm water or ginger tea before bed.

Thyme (*Thymus vulgaris*)

Parts used: *Leaves and flowering tops*

Thyme is rich in essential oils that provide potent antimicrobial, antispasmodic, expectorant, and diaphoretic properties. It has traditionally been used as an antiseptic and for alleviating indigestion and coughs.

A hot infusion of thyme tea helps to loosen mucous congestion in the respiratory tract and relieves spasmodic coughs. Thyme can also be used as a steam inhalation to cleanse the sinuses and lungs of excess mucus, while the antimicrobial action helps to fight bacteria and viruses in the respiratory tract. A cup of thyme tea after meals eases indigestion and intestinal gas.

Thyme has a pleasantly spicy flavor. To make a thyme tea, pour 1 cup of boiling water over 1 to 2 teaspoons of dried thyme and steep for 10 minutes. Strain, and drink up to 3 cups a day. To use thyme as an herbal steam inhalation, pour 1 1/2 quarts of boiling water over 4 tablespoons of dried thyme. Cover, and let steep for 10 minutes. Make a towel tent over your head and the bowl of steaming water and inhale the steam for 10 minutes, taking care to not burn yourself with the steam.

Turmeric (*Curcuma longa*)

Part used: *Root*

Turmeric has been valued in Ayurvedic medicine for centuries as a whole body cleansing herb. It has natural antimicrobial properties, and is used to strengthen digestion and to improve the health of beneficial intestinal flora. Turmeric has powerful antioxidant properties as well as a variety of other health-promoting benefits. It protects the body against the formation of carcinogens, and also enhances levels of glutathione, one of the most potent natural antioxidants produced by the body. Turmeric has been shown to inhibit cancer, and may even help to promote the regression of existing cancers.

Turmeric also has beneficial effects on the cardiovascular system. It blocks the absorption of cholesterol in the intestinal tract, helping to lower levels of blood cholesterol. In addition, it prevents the clumping together of blood cells that contributes to atherosclerosis. The antioxidant action of turmeric protects the liver against toxins and the bitter components stimulate liver cleansing by enhancing bile production.

Turmeric appears to be best absorbed when taken with meals containing fats. In traditional Ayurvedic medicine, turmeric is taken in warm milk, 1 teaspoon of powdered turmeric stirred into 1 cup of milk. Because cow's milk often causes congestion or allergies, try taking turmeric in soy milk if the traditional Ayurvedic recipe appeals to you. Turmeric can also be used liberally in cooking, in curries, soups, and grain dishes, and it can be taken in capsule form with meals.

Uva Ursi (*Arctostaphylos uva-ursi*)

Part used: *Leaves*

Uva ursi, also called *bearberry*, has antimicrobial, astringent, diuretic, and antiseptic properties that specifically act on the urinary system. It contains a natural chemical that is transformed into a potent antiseptic in the urinary tract. Uva ursi has been used for centuries by Chinese herbalists and by Native Americans to relieve kidney and bladder problems. It is especially helpful for bladder infections, and if taken at the first sign of discomfort (usually urinary urgency, frequent urination, or burning upon urination) can help to prevent a full-blown infection. Do not attempt to self-treat a kidney infection. If you have symptoms such as fever, blood in the urine, or pain in the kidney region, immediately consult your health care practitioner for advice.

Uva ursi has an astringent taste. To make a tea, pour 1 cup of boiling water over 1 to 2 teaspoons of dried leaves and steep for 10 minutes. Strain, and drink 4 cups throughout the day when treating a bladder infection. To relieve burning urination, uva ursi can be combined with soothing diuretic herbs such as cornsilk or marshmallow root. Because it works best in an alkaline environment, avoid acidic foods such as citrus fruits and cranberries while using uva ursi.

Yarrow (*Achillea millefolium*)

Parts used: *Flowers, leaves, and stems*

Yarrow has been used for thousands of years by many cultures. The ancient Chinese used yarrow to stop bleeding, including heavy menstrual bleeding, and to soothe inflammations. Ayurvedic physicians in India prescribed yarrow to reduce fevers. The astringent and antiseptic properties found in yarrow make it helpful for treating cuts, wounds, hemorrhoids, and as a vaginal wash for leukorrhea. Yarrow tea is also useful used as a urinary antiseptic to relieve cystitis.

Natural chemicals in yarrow have anti-inflammatory, antispasmodic, and pain-relieving properties, which help to ease menstrual cramps and to relax the digestive tract. In addition, the bitter taste of yarrow makes it useful as a mild digestive stimulant. Yarrow is one of the most effective diaphoretic herbs. It contains a high concentration of volatile oils which stimulate circulation, encouraging sweating and the elimination of toxins through the skin. Hot yarrow tea is excellent for treating a cold or flu. It stimulates the body to naturally raise a fever, which helps to kill off the invading microorganisms.

Yarrow has a slightly bitter and astringent flavor. Make an infusion by steeping 1 to 2 teaspoons of dried herb in 1 cup of boiling water for 10 to 15 minutes. Strain, and drink up to 3 cups daily. Yarrow combines well with peppermint and elder flower as a tea for colds and flus. Blend equal parts of yarrow and chamomile for a gentle digestive tea. An infusion of yarrow can be used externally as a skin wash to heal cuts and wounds, or as a sponge bath to bring down a fever. To relieve vaginal infections or hemorrhoids, add a quart of strong yarrow tea to a warm sitz bath.

Yellow Dock (*Rumex crispus*)

Part used: *Root*

Yellow dock has long been regarded as a classic blood-cleansing herb. The bitter taste of yellow dock stimulates the flow of bile and helps to naturally cleanse the liver. This creates a gentle laxative effect, which is helpful for alleviating sluggish bowels or chronic constipation. It gently restores proper bowel function without the use of strong purgatives. Because of its action on clearing toxins from the blood and intestinal tract, yellow dock is often recommended for the treatment of skin problems such as eczema, psoriasis, boils, and other skin eruptions. It is rich in iron and helps to build healthy blood.

Make a decoction by simmering 1 teaspoon of dried root in 1 cup of water for 15 minutes. Strain, and drink up to 3 cups daily. Yellow dock is bitter and tastes best if combined with sweet and spicy herbs such as licorice, fennel, or ginger. As a blood cleanser, yellow dock is traditionally used with other liver-cleansing herbs such as burdock, Oregon grape root, or sarsaparilla.

Resources

Alternative Health Practitioners

American Association of Acupuncture and Oriental Medicine
4101 Lake Boone Trail, Suite 201
Raleigh, NC 27607
(919) 787-5181

American Association of Naturopathic Physicians
2366 Eastlake Avenue, Suite 322
Seattle, WA 98102
(206) 323-7610

American Holistic Medical Association
4101 Lake Boone Trail, Suite 201
Raleigh, NC 27607
(919) 787-5181

Ayurvedic Institute
11311 Menaul N.E., Suite A
Albuquerque, NM 87112
(505) 291-9698

Aromatherapy

National Association for Holistic Aromatherapy
219 Carl Street
San Francisco, CA 94117

Reference Books:

The Encyclopedia of Essential Oils, by Julia Lawless
(Element, 1992)

Aromatherapy: A Complete Guide to the Healing Art, by Kathi
Keville and Mindy Green
(The Crossing Press, 1995)

Mail-Order Essential Oils:

Prima Fleur Botanicals
1201-R Anderson Dr.
San Rafael, CA 94901
(415) 455-0956

Simpler's Botanical Co.
P. O. Box 39
Forestville, CA 95436

Healthy Home

Reference books:

Nontoxic, Natural, and Earthwise, by Debra Lynn Dadd
(Tarcher, 1990)

Mail-order catalogues:

Seventh Generation
49 Hercules Drive
Colchester, VT 05446
(800) 456-1177

The Natural Choice
1365 Rufina Circle
Santa Fe, NM 87505
(800) 621-2591

Herbs

Reference books:

Identifying and Harvesting Edible and Medicinal Plants, by Steve Brill
(Hearst Books, 1994)

The Complete Illustrated Holistic Herbal, by David Hoffmann
(Element, 1996)

Herbs for Health and Healing, by Kathi Keville
(Rodale Press, 1996)

Herbal Healing for Women, by Rosemary Gladstar
(Fireside, 1993)

The Herbs of Life, by Lesley Tierra
(The Crossing Press, 1992)

Mail-Order Herbs:

Mountain Rose Herbs
P. O. Box 2000
Redway, CA 95560
(800) 879-3337

Witch Hazel and Broom
258 "A" Street
Ashland, OR 97520
(541) 482-9628

Mail-Order Natural Foods

Diamond Organics
Freedom, CA 95019
(888) 674-2642

Mountain Ark Trading Company
120 South East Avenue
Fayetteville, AR 72701
(800) 643-8909

Natural Lifestyles Supplies
16 Lookout Drive
Asheville, NC 28804
(704) 254-9606

Massage

American Massage Therapy Association
820 Davis Street, Suite 100
Evanston, IL 60201
(312) 761-2682

Reference books and video:

The Book of Massage, by Lucinda Lidell
(Fireside, 1984)

The Book of Shiatsu, by Paul Lundberg
(Fireside, 1992)

Massage for Health
(Healing Arts Home Video)

Natural Bodycare Products

Reference books for making your own:

The Herbal Body Book, by Stephanie Tourles
(Storey Publishing, 1994)

The Essential Oils Book, by Colleen Dodt
(Storey Publishing, 1996)

Natural Healing and Home Remedies

Natural Health Magazine
17 Station Street
Brookline, MA 02146

The Complete Home Healer, by Angela Smyth
(Harper San Francisco, 1994)

Dr. Whitaker's Guide to Natural Healing, by Julian Whitaker, M.D.
(Prima, 1995)

Natural Alternatives to Over-the-Counter and Prescription Drugs,
by Michael Murray, N.D.
(Morrow, 1994)

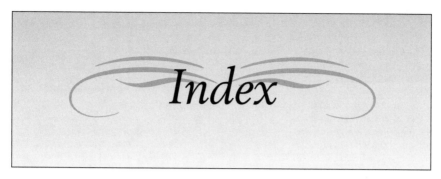

Index